*A Record of the Assembled Immortals and
Gathered Perfected of the Western Hills*

by the same author

The Great Intent
Acupuncture Odes, Songs and Rhymes
Richard Bertschinger
ISBN 978 1 84819 132 7
eISBN 978 0 85701 111 4

The Secret of Everlasting Life
The First Translation of the Ancient
Chinese Text on Immortality
Richard Bertschinger
ISBN 978 1 84819 048 1
eISBN 978 0 85701 054 4

Yijing, Shamanic Oracle of China
A New Book of Change
Translated with commentary by Richard Bertschinger
ISBN 978 1 84819 083 2
eISBN 978 0 85701 066 7

Everyday Qigong Practice
Richard Bertschinger
Illustrated by Harriet E.J. Lewars
ISBN 978 1 84819 117 4
eISBN 978 0 85701 097 1

Essential Texts in Chinese Medicine
The Single Idea in the Mind of the Yellow Emperor
Richard Bertschinger
ISBN 978 1 84819 162 4
eISBN 978 0 85701 135 0

of related interest

The Way of the Five Seasons
Living with the Five Elements for Physical,
Emotional, and Spiritual Harmony
John Kirkwood
ISBN 978 1 84819 301 7
eISBN 978 0 85701 252 4

Daoist Meditation
The Purification of the Heart Method of Meditation and Discourse
on Sitting and Forgetting (Zuò Wàng Lùn) by Si Ma Cheng Zhen
Translated and with a commentary by Wu Jyh Cherng
ISBN 978 1 84819 211 9
eISBN 978 0 85701 161 9

A Record of the Assembled Immortals and Gathered Perfected of the Western Hills

Shi Jianwu's Daoist Classic on Internal Alchemy and the Cultivation of the Breath

RICHARD BERTSCHINGER

Foreword by Master Zhongxian Wu

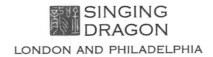
SINGING
DRAGON
LONDON AND PHILADELPHIA

First published in 2018
by Singing Dragon
an imprint of Jessica Kingsley Publishers
73 Collier Street
London N1 9BE, UK
and
400 Market Street, Suite 400
Philadelphia, PA 19106, USA

www.singingdragon.com

Library of Congress Cataloging in Publication Data
A CIP catalog record for this book is available from the Library of Congress

British Library Cataloguing in Publication Data
A CIP catalogue record for this book is available from the British Library

ISBN 978 1 84819 387 1
eISBN 978 0 85701 344 6

Printed and bound in Great Britain

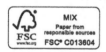

To the three sages of Emei Mountain...

I'm going back to the old home,
Back to the home I love so well.
Where the sweet waters flow
And the wild flowers grow,
All around the old home on the hill.

Doc Watson

This is why the sage puts on rough clothing while holding the jewel in his heart.

Tao-te Ching

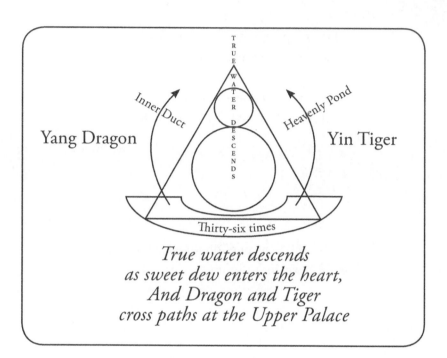

Yang Dragon   Yin Tiger

True water descends
as sweet dew enters the heart,
And Dragon and Tiger
cross paths at the Upper Palace

Contents

Foreword

THE IMMORTALS' MESSAGES

Master Zhongxian Wu

Shi JianWu 施肩吾 (780–861 CE), who is also known by his Daoist names, XiZhenZi 棲真子 and HuaYangZhenRen 華陽真人, was a famous Daoist scholar, prolific author and cultivation practitioner from the Tang 唐 Dynasty. An astounding number of his poems were showcased in *QuanTangShi* 全唐詩 (*Complete Tang Poems*). Commissioned by the Qing Emperor himself, the *QuanTangShi* is the largest compilation of Tang poetry to date. Whilst most of the poets represented in this publication had only a few works chosen, this anthology memorialised 197 of Shi JianWu's poems. An exceptional human being, Shi JianWu passed up opportunities for the great power and wealth enjoyed by the highest-ranking government officials of the time, becoming one of the rare exceptions of Chinese history – a person who prioritised his personal cultivation above all else.

Of all the Daoist classics, I personally believe his work, *XiShanQunXianHuiZhenJi* 西山群仙會真記 (*A True Record of the Assembled Immortals of the Western Hills*), is amongst the best practical texts on internal alchemy and Qigong cultivation.

In the original preface, HuaYangZhenRen states that he deliberately wrote this book in five volumes in order to represent the numerological energy of WuXing 五行 (Five Elements). Each volume contains five chapters, which together represent one pure YangQi 炁 of each of the Five Elements (in other words, in five there is one).

He also asserts that whilst 'everyone' knows WuXing and the related birth and controlling principles, only a rare few know how to apply these principles to enter the Dao 道. Whilst 'everyone' also knows the three DanTian 丹田 and their associations with the Three Layers of JingQiShen 精炁神, scarcely any know how to circulate them through the three DanTian in order to attain the Dao. From my experience in the Qigong and Daoist cultivation world, I am astonished how little has changed in the last 1200 years!

The teachings of this book are a true treasure trove for the Daoist practitioner. Drawing from cryptic messages of old Daoist masters, the *CanTongQi* 參同契 (reputed as the king of internal alchemy classics), and the *ZhongLu DanFa* 鐘呂丹法 (the internal alchemy techniques of Daoist immortals ZhongLiQuan 鐘離權 and LuDongBing 呂洞賓), Shi JianWu particularly emphasises the key inner cultivation methods of WuXing and the three DanTian. By doing so, he reminds us of the most essential (and most often overlooked) elements of the Daoist cultivation tradition and modern Qigong practices.

I welcome the birth of the English version of this important internal alchemy classic with enthusiasm! Guided by Richard Bertschinger's expert translation and annotations, I hope many people will gain great benefits from this vital work.

A Short Note on
Reading the Text

There are two distinct ways of reading these dense spiritual texts: one is quicker, to let the strange words and passages wash over you – without too much thinking what they mean; the other is slower, letting the significance of each phrase resonate in the brain, sparking involvement and depth of feeling. Both are fine, and both okay. Think of it as approaching a banquet – some dishes to be savoured, others consumed with their accompanying sauces and condiments easing their passage. You are literally 'munching meaning'. Here is a summary of the highlights.

The first section explains the historical context of this remarkable method of softening the breath. Chapter 1 explains the One Path, the Dao, and is fairly self-explanatory. Chapter 2 tells us that it all hinges on 'acting naturally'. Simply marry together both forms of breathing, the True Yin and Proper Yang, and it is then possible to form an inner Medicine. Chapter 3 explains how to secure this elixial ('health-giving') method – essentially not to make too much of it, but to remain peacefully and inwardly content without striving. Chapter 4 speaks of timing this action, along with the turning over of the natural world – the crux of the affair. This is our task – to silently join 'in fit accord' with Yin and Yang, smelting out the True Yin and Yang in the body. This chapter contains the first mention of 'sustaining' – that is, sustaining the Yin and Yang of all life. Chapter 5 continues to elaborate on the same theme – extracting the True Yin and Yang breaths.

The second section describes further 'the sustaining'. This means sustaining the True Yin and Yang. Chapter 6 explains sustaining life through the quiet withdrawal of the body, and the physical senses. The *Zhouyi Cantong Qi* concludes: 'the ear, the eye and mouth, these three jewels, block and stop them up, do not let them gape.'[1] Chapters 7 and 8 continue the same theme. Chapter 9 emphasises 'uncluttering the heart'. The final chapter, Chapter 10, points us towards our ultimate goal – 'walking in the divine'.

The next section is on rebuilding – that is, rebuilding our physical health, fluid-essences, vital breaths, spirit, etc. Chapter 11 is specifically on rebuilding the body's internal form, and sustaining its five main internal breaths. Chapters 12, 13 and 14 are also on rebuilding and strengthening the five internal organs (*zang*). In Chapter 15 an additional method is given, using the sound, and voicing certain common words, or sounds, under the breath – the 'method of the Six Character Breaths' – meaning there is sound for each of the main organs. These activities further strengthen the breath.

The penultimate section does no more than verify this remarkable technique. Chapters 16–19 elaborate previously described practices, giving the detail. They describe especial 'alchemic happenings' in the body, the merging of the True Yin (fluid) and Proper Yang (breath), forming a state of so-called 'perfection'. Chapter 20 identifies the end of the quest, a quiet and gentle form of 'foetal breath', as if we were still a foetus in our mother's tummy, breathing out as our mother breathes out and breathing in as she breathes in. This is the highest achievement we are able to attain in this 'dusty world'. It fits and fortifies us with its Great Simplicity.

The last section in the book is on refining the technique. It is achieved through making quiet and settled times during the day to work on the breath. This should be practised at regular intervals, times set aside for just being with the practice. Good luck!

---

1   See Chapter 25 in my translation of this foundation text, *The Secret of Everlasting Life* (Singing Dragon, 2012).

INTRODUCTION

As I sit back and think about this old text on internal alchemy, I experience afresh the wonder I felt when first deciphering its characters, crouched in a field on the edge of Exmoor, alone on one of my weekend hikes. I remember the astonishment I felt at its clear exposition of Daoist meditation practice and its denigration of unorthodox techniques; its philosophical pairing of sun and moon, the organic duo, the rhythm of Yin and the Yang; the exquisite imagery and simple instruction; the intricate diagrams (of my own creation), illustrating traditional Chinese medicine and an almost arcane approach to the health arts: a picture of the interpenetration of macrocosm and microcosm, the True Breath, Five Elements, water and fire, the human and divine, and much more besides. Its roots go back to the philosophy of the Dao. 'Dao' can be variously translated as 'Way' or 'Path', and is described well in the seminal *Tao-te Ching*, foundation text of the Daoists, a motley crew of hermits, proto-chemists, recuperative physicians and great naturalists born in China around 200 BCE to 200 CE.

Crouched as I was in that Exmoor field, I pored over the characters, and immediately on getting home retreated to my study to complete the translation. It was finished in a few weeks – and needed little revision. Surrounded by the gentle hills of the West Country, there was an undeniable affinity with those seers of Western China. In my copy of old *Zhuangzi*,[1] a section on the 'hearts of the ancients' explains how the sincerity and integrity of the one searching for meaning in these texts may reveal a true affinity of souls, how

---

1 Zhuangzi was a pivotal fourth-century BCE Daoist philosopher.

the hearts of the ancient and the present may easily and graciously become one.

This small book is dated around 820 CE, the heyday of Mahayana Buddhism in China, and was written by the Daoist practitioner Shi Jianwu (780–861 CE). He was a prominent figure in the ancient and by then thoroughly tangled so-called Zhong-Lu (鍾呂) tradition of internal alchemy (*neidan*), or self-cultivation.[2] This book rendered a clear account of how to acquire and develop the so-called 'astral body', the goal of much Daoist and Buddhist practice. I found it lodged in a large compendium of historical texts[3] on 'nourishing life' (*yangsheng*) recently published in China. This volume was the one single copy left on the shelf. Shi Jianwu's work caught my notice immediately – because of its brevity of style.

It broke into five main sections: the knowledge, or rediscovering the balance of Yin and Yang; the sustaining of their breath-energy in our bodies – or 'inner laboratory'; the rebuilding, as perhaps we might have been already been weakened; the verification or crux of the affair; and, finally, the refinement, whereby we learn to acquire another body – and move from our physical existence to 'walk in the divine'.

These few steps were carefully set out – with tales and stories told 'along the way', to enlighten and encourage the practitioner. The ultimate aim was to create a 'higher self'. I was gripped. It seemed to be the key to spiritual transformation. The Chinese had discovered the inner true breath as the key to transforming the human soul.

In pre-internet days, Chinese texts were hard to get. It was during one of my forays into Chinatown, just north of Leicester Square, that I had come across Shi Jianwu. With his poetic style he took

---

2   Shi Jianwu's most famous two works are the *Zhong-Lü Chuandaoji* (*Records of the Transmission of the Dao from Zhongli Quan to Lü Dongbin*) and the work in question, the *Xishan Qunxian Huizhen Ji* (*A True Record of the Assembled Immortals of the Western Hills*).

3   Fang, Chunyang 方春陽 ed. 1992. *The Great Anthology of Chinese Nourishing Life Studies*, Zhongguo Yangsheng Dacheng 中國养生大成. Jiling: Jiling Science and Technology Press.

me deep into the spiritual heart of the Chinese people. Here we are informed that the Himalayan sages set down a record of how to reach inner peace, worked on the five internal organs (heart, liver, lungs, spleen and kidneys), and tuned in to the season of the year, sounding and softening the breath. Along with this, they tell of a spiritual dimension, an astral self that may escape our fleshly existence ('shed the husk'), and lead into the ranks of the Immortals.

As I carried this book back to my house in Essex, there was a great feeling in my heart, as if I had come 'back home' – for somehow I had known the truth of this all for a long time. It was as if I was privy to a great and comforting understanding.

The remarkably large and valuable volume I had in my bag contained a great many original works from the Chinese long-life tradition. Texts from the ancient Han tombs, erudite studies of *daoyin*, sexology and meditation from the Tang and Song dynasties, and, later, more leisurely written essays and summaries penned by Qing scholars. The wealth and range of material was fascinating.

But Shi Jianwu's discussion stood out. At that time, I had largely finished the *Zhouyi Cantong Qi* (*Combining Similars Together and the Changes of Zhou*, the grand-daddy of all alchemical works); I had a working copy or two of my translation of the *Kangxi Yijing* (the imperial compendium compiled in 1715), and had just completed my work on Zhang Boduan's *Wuzhen Pian* (*Understanding the Truth about Reality*), along with his shorter works.[4] I had previously taken a degree in Philosophy, spent some time in teaching, and had made an in-depth study of traditional acupuncture, after many years' experience of meditation, tai chi and the rest – from Hare Krishna to 'Have-a-go Joe' yoga at the local college evening classes! I am glad, so glad now, nearly 60 years later, to see it all bearing some sort of fruit.

---

4   The first is published as *The Secret of Everlasting Life* (Singing Dragon, 2011), the second as *Yijing, Shamanic Oracle of China* (Singing Dragon, 2012), and the third self-published as *Written upon Awakening to Reality: A Translation of Zhang Boduan's Guide to Internal Alchemy* (CreateSpace, 2016).

Shi Jianwu's work is entitled *A True Record of the Assembled Immortals of the Western Hills* (*Xishan Qunxian Huizhen Ji* 西山群仙會真記). He unites together three subjects: traditional Chinese medical theory, with its emphasis on 'joining and connecting' Yin and Yang and the Five Elements (*wuxing*); the trigram symbolism of the anciently reconstructed *Yijing*; and lastly, the Daoist guiding principle of *tianren heyi* 天人合一, or 'oneness of heaven and humankind'. This is the belief that we are all, every single one of us, an integral part of nature – although we also have individual strengths and abilities, enough, that is, to reach a very supra-divine, immortal existence, in this so-human life.

Whilst Shi Jianwu was writing, Daoist thinking existed as a hotch-potch of beliefs in spirits, gods, fairies and other faculties, lumped in with healthcare practices (meditation, therapeutic exercise, *daoyin* or massage, qigong, etc.); a deep fascination with all nature and life; and attempts to explain the biological and physical prowess of the teeming profusion of the world (*huntun* 混沌). In his last few paragraphs the writer celebrates with an admonition to truly believe in and to spread this knowledge, in the correct manner. All these factors drew me to this work.

Each of its five sections contains five chapters – Shi Jianwu reads like a dream. His text gives clear instruction in how to nurture the breath, strengthen the internal organs of the body and refine the spirit.

It aims to lay to rest all delusions by focusing on breathing naturally, along with the round of the year and turn of the day. Much of this it is easy to forget, and get wrong! A few years previously I had been lucky and met Gia-fu Feng (1919–1985), who drove me to read and re-read these Chinese classics, and he explained how, in the ten years I studied with him, to take a first few steps on the Path. Then I visited China, during the 1980s, the year after he died. Certainly much had been destroyed and gone, but much was still the same, and being rediscovered. I found a living tradition, which involved the cultivation of a gentle breath, and dedicate this small book to the unnamed I met there in Sichuan province, living on Qingcheng Shan ('Green City Mountain').

I have always had a thing about mountains. I was born on the clays and gravels of the Stort Valley, in Essex, southern England, and it was not until I was eight or nine that I saw mountains for real. I remember well, peering out of the car windows of our new Ford Consul Estate on the way to Switzerland and the annual 'family holiday'. Later I was to get to know the isolated areas around Deborance in the Canton de Valais region, and here felt an affinity with its precipitous screes and unstable peaks, and in 1986, when I spent nearly a week on Qingcheng Mountain, I found it redolent, in fact stuffed with Daoist tales and hagiographies. Two other places: an area of Central Wales, of old flat, denuded, Silurian sands and mudstones, where I met a true Lama from Tibet; and also the time I returned three consecutive winters to Stillpoint Hermitage, Colorado, in the young Rockies, close to the Sangre de Cristo Range, when I worked and studied with Gia-fu Feng. He was Shanghai-born but had been enlivened by the Californian exodus of the early 1970s. His *Tao-te Ching*, with Jane English's memorable black-and-white photos, still lingers.

The Song poet, artist and statesman Su Dongpo (also known as Su Shi, 1037–1101) famously said, 'Wherever you are living, let your eyes rise up to the hills.' No wonder the great mountain system of Asia, the Himalayas ('dwelling of the snows'), was the birthplace of the deepest wisdom of mankind. Shi Jianwu records this wisdom, of a breath that unites and strengthens mind and body, releasing a higher spirit – variously called many things, but, in essence, the astral body, or greater self ('outside the body, there is a body'). The merit of his work is that it is packed with stories and tales of Daoist exploits and forays into these *yangsheng* ('health-giving') practices. They yield explicit instruction in the physical techniques of acquiring a higher 'soul'. But his point is that we need to cultivate physical health first – worrying about finer matters afterwards. This is a shining example of the dual cultivation of both body and mind, the genius of Daoist practice.

From their earliest days, Daoist texts (for instance, the Heshang Gong commentary on the *Tao-te Ching*[5]) involved physical exertion: body and breath together in harmonious accord. Spirituality could involve a physio-logical approach; it was not just logical. Throughout the centuries, Daoist authors would describe fairly accurately how they were changing their body's own neurochemistry and higher cortical functioning; some might contest they could alter their own DNA (*xing*).[6]

Shi Jianwu's genius is that he keeps it all relatively simple. As I have stressed previously,[7] the acute sensibility of the old Chinese is a very tangible thing, 'in your face' and alive. It engages our 'sensory logic', touching every part of the body. The activity of our simian frontal cortex, an object of fascination in the West, often seems as an obstacle to the oriental – indeed, 'Give up learning and put an end to your troubles!' (*Tao-te Ching*, Ch.22).

I remember walking across Holkham beach, after my first few days spend with Gia-fu, in north Norfolk, very confused in mind… when I finally caught up with him, I broke the silence: 'Please can you help me, the trouble with the *Yijing*, you see, is that sometimes I understand, and sometimes I don't.' He swung round and looked me straight in the eyes, 'That's it! Don't understand!' I must say, I certainly did not see what he was getting at here. What did he mean? Not to understand? But the fierceness of his manner was utterly convincing. His intervention left me reeling.

Well, one way of getting closer to the meaning of this encounter might be by attempting to solve the riddle set in Lao Zi's *Tao-te Ching*, Chapter 71. This tortuous text fascinated me whilst I was at the Needham Research Institute in 1986. The great man himself

---

5   Available from my website as *Treasuries of the Tao* (self-published), at http://mytaoworld.com

6   *Xing* is usually rendered nature, but also has the sense of that stamp that makes each of us unique.

7   See my Introduction to *Essential Texts in Chinese Medicine: The Single Idea in the Mind of the Yellow Emperor* (Singing Dragon, 2014).

(Professor Joseph Needham) had a large calligraphic wall hanging of this chapter hanging outside his room: 'Be wrong about being wrong, then you are not wrong...the sage is wrong about being wrong, so he is not wrong.'

The whole passage actually reads:

> To know that you do not know is best. Not to know, but to think you know – is just plain wrong. Only be wrong about being wrong. Then you will not be wrong. The clever man is not wrong, because he is wrong about being wrong. So he is not wrong.[8]

What is clear here is that Lao Zi sees 'being wrong' as the human disease. To know that you do not know is best. The 'clever man' is the 'sage'. He is able to trust his gut feeling. It is the thinking that gets us into trouble. Presumably we need to trust to something more like instinct; perhaps it is ancestral, our inborn human nature, vis-à-vis the 'common or garden' DNA.

Again, this is the point. 'Yin and Yang' mean there are often two ways (at least!) of looking at things. As we understand, being no way uncertain yet retaining a humility of position – of quiet and stillness – the Path may be found:

> A humble heart banishes all fullness.
> A vacant heart is redolent with life.
> At the still-point without stirring,
> We become settled and immune from danger.[9]

And again, 'The True method involves nothing else than being at peace within, and not labouring at the work.'

It is at moments such as this that we simply know, and understand. It is not a reasoned position – but neither is it fundamentalist. Let us call it fundamentalism with a small 'f'. There is a distinct lack of force, with no wish to rush into action. We remain 'gently at anchor,

---

8   知不知上；不知知病。夫唯病病，是以不病。聖人不病，以其病病，
     是以不病，I translate *bing* as 'wrong', rather than the more common 'sick'.

9   From Chapter 9 (p.38).

peaceful and calm, trusting in the Path for our preservation'.[10] In existential terms, this is our 'centre', representative of both true happiness and humanness (the Confucian virtue *ren*). I believe Shi Jianwu is telling us to simply be – and to be gentle.

He quotes much from the original *Western Mountain Records*, many now lost to fire, flood and decay. But he also draws on sayings (often remembered orally) by well-recognised figures. Bodhidharma, the Indian Buddhist monk in his *Supreme Method of the Foetal Breath*, is quoted as saying, 'If we allow our breath to rise upwards, we are lost.' Here Shi Jianwu pointedly comments: 'There is no better practice, in his view, than the inner gazing of the several worlds, that we may amuse ourselves playing in the Hall of Heaven, and escape into the clear void and Place of All Mysteries.' In this case, I think his tongue was firmly in his cheek.

But he also mentions the historical figure of Bian Que (fourth century BCE) and his commentary on the *Spiritual Pivot* (the *Lingshu* section of the *Huangdi Neijing*):

> ...when it came to the time just after the winter solstice, when a fraction of the 'true lead' accumulates within the body, shaped like a 'sporting stamen', he crushed it down into his *dantian*, instructing his people to use the nose to guide in the clean air, to close up the mouth and not let the breath out.

He also includes the famous Daoist researcher Ge Hong, who commented in his *Discourse on the Foetal Breath*, 'generally this "foetal breath" has one crucial distinction; it is as if held in your mother's belly...as your mother breathes out, so you breathe out, as your mother breathes in, so you breathe in.'

This strange work from a distant land, and foreign heart, tells us of the deeply mystical centre within each of us – speaking of the similarities of human souls, regardless of creed, nationality, ethnicity, sex, colour, etc. It gives each of us an opportunity to reach up, up,

---

10   From the commentary to 'Nine at the Second' in Hexagram 10 *Stepping* of the *Yijing*.

as 'the true water descends', until we join in the resplendent spiritual brother- or sisterhood of 'attained immortals' – the 'gold eternal', as in the Christian 'New Jerusalem' or Buddhist 'nirvana'.[11] It can rank alongside the medieval 'Pearl', written by the Gawain poet with its vision of a New Jerusalem. *In Tune with the Infinite* by Ralph Waldo Trine, *Revelations of Divine Love* by Dame Julian, or even the twin works of Pseudo-Dionysius, *The Celestial Hierarchy* and *Mystical Theology*. But enough of false analogies! Here in your hand you hold one of the treasures of world literature: read, practise, and enjoy.

Outside my window seventeen geese are now flying over the wooded St Michael's Hill, in this ancient English village. Are these the seventeen souls of Daoist monks come to surprise me from the Tang dynasty? I suspect so. It has been a struggle somewhat to complete the work, and I need their support! As far as I can ascertain, the book contains a true record of those immortal folk who lived in seclusion on the slopes of the Himalayas in early ninth-century China. But meditation needs practice. If you want to eat the rice, you have to cook it! I would encourage you to find a teacher. There is much to comment on in the alchemical world.

Master Zhongxian Wu has agreed to write a foreword to this work, and I am enormously grateful – he has also helped in so many other ways, quite immeasurable. I must also thank Jessica Kingsley and her superlative team for their inexhaustible effort.

Richard, Somerset, August 2017

---

11 Admittedly, nirvana has a greater sense of 'extinguishment'.

The Knowledge

1

Knowing the Path

...there can never be two Paths...

THERE HAS ONLY EVERY BEEN ONE PATH THROUGHOUT all times and ages. Yet how greatly it does dissemble into so many views, opinions and schools! So says our Gentleman Immortal.

> *NOTE: There has only ever been One Path. At the beginning the author draws on the sayings of Ge Hong (Gentleman Immortal), his spiritual teacher. It is in the nature of the self to bring completion and dispense a single truth; the former Sages were all in essence preserving One Mind. Achieving this single mind and through it dispensing the True Breath is our goal.*

There can never be two Paths – there may be varying tracks, but they all end up at the same place. In similar fashion the Sages themselves were never in doubt in their hearts about anything: all their ideas pursued a single goal.

From time immemorial there has always existed One Path, and the saints and sages have all been of one mind.

But once the Path and source divides, the mind's understanding also splits into two, and any discussion does violence to its true nature. It fragments apart: the single flow dividing into differing streams, from the root arising leaves and branches; then, of their own accord, arise differing views and opinions, standing alone and apart as differing sects and Schools.

The pattern of the ten-thousand things can never be exhausted, for once the true nature of the single self dawns there comes harmony and completion. For instance, the Buddhists talk of the wayward Void, and subsequently from this present world look towards a latter one, whilst the Confucians look at where they are, and then those of lesser years pay their respects to those older than them. But these people never actually realise that the former Sages were actually walking One Path and preserving, in essence, One Mind.

THE *WESTERN MOUNTAIN RECORDS* STATE: WHEN Teacher Lu spoke out, as he was young he spoke as a Confucian scholar, but when older he loved to model himself on the teachings of our true self-nature.

> To cultivate the dignity of Heaven
> And reject that conferred by Man.
> To despise the greedy and empty
> And awaken to the True Void.

For Heaven's dignity rests ultimately in the present, in human affairs – whilst the True Void of the Daoists is no different from the Buddhist's chain of cause and effect.

Our Gentleman Immortal has said: Take the Five Constants to describe the Way, and you probably find yourself a few remnants; make use of the Three Religions to view your own self-nature, and in a cumbersome manner you can peer at its roots and main stalk.

But the fact is that the Confucians and Buddhists are all swept along in this single Great Path; throughout ten thousand generations, the fellow who has pursued this knowledge has always set his or her soul upon a quiet humility and attention to the Silent Source.

NOTE: Truly a knowledge of the Way is not encompassed
by any of the main three religions of China: Confucianism,
Buddhism or Daoism. The attitude is one of quiet humility,
which is reached by attending to the Silent Source, a
fountain of originating power that donates us life. The
Five Constants are water, fire, wood, earth and metal.

But how has this happened? Beginning from the settled joy of preserving his years, our friend has attained an unfailing old age; he has secretly stolen away the clue to the Workings of Heaven, that he then may apply them to himself!

Thenceforth from being human he has ascended and discovered life as an Immortal, finding his very place in the Temple of Heaven; how could merely being a good Confucian have done this? One hundred winters he is working and he attains one thousand years! Is this the same as the case of a Buddhist monk who is recompensed in a latter world, in the nirvana hereafter?

If you want to foster and sustain this truth, you must distinguish whole-heartedly between the right and wrong methods. If you desire to know the correct Path, then place our great Lord Lao Zi, father of them all, as foremost. What need then do you have of seeking beyond the confines of your own body and self!

2

法

Knowing the Method

...to join silently in fit accord with the rise and fall of
all things, and to display the general rule of Yin and
Yang, the coming and going of the sun and moon, the
Hun and Po-souls.

THE METHOD IS NONE OTHER THAN THE METHOD
that appears as *no method*, none other than the method of acting
naturally. This is an idea attributed to *The Secret Book of Our Father*
(Lao Zi).

When the heart is relied upon at the borders of confusion, the
method is none other than that which is born within the heart.

NOTE: The method is none other than no significant method.
It rests in simply being oneself, in non-action, and responding
from the heart. This is where Buddhism and Daoism merge;
our self-nature is our original 'face and eyes'. The phrase 'at
the borders of confusion' expresses the state of the novice, or
beginner. The method will be born on its own within the
innocent heart, through steadfast practice. Thus the true
method is none other than acting simply and being constant.
This is to practise in accord with the course of the Dao.

The significance of establishing a method is that a method can rescue that which has already been lost, and guard against that which has not yet been lost. As a consequence of this, all the three thousand and six hundred methods of sustaining life fall into ten categories.

> *NOTE: There are many, many schools of sustaining and*
> *cultivating life. The author will now proceed to categorise*
> *and list several of them. Lastly he will dispense with them*
> *all – to assert his own simple practice of marrying the breath.*

These three thousand and six hundred methods all fall into ten families. There are three thousand and six hundred because they cover a term of ten years. The methods of sustaining life are numbered into ten families – Heaven-one, earth-two, Heaven-three, earth-four, Heaven-five, earth-six, Heaven-seven, earth-eight, Heaven-nine, earth-ten. One, three, five, seven and nine are the Yang numbers of the cycle; two, four, six, eight and ten are the Yin numbers of the cycle.

The Great Path splits and becomes Two Breaths; the Two Breaths divide to become the Five Cycles of Form. Their majesty lies in the fact that they create Heaven and earth, their brilliance lies in the sun and moon, their magic lies in man.

There is nothing in existence not actually endowed with these Two Breaths, giving birth to the Five Cycles of Form. Everything travels through the Five Cycles, implicating the Three Powers of Heaven, earth and Man.

> *NOTE: This is the Way of the Great Golden Elixir*
> *incorporating the Two Breaths of Yin and Yang,*
> *which endow all things with life. The Five Cycles of*
> *Form are the passages of wood, earth, fire, metal and*
> *water. Majestically they create Heaven and earth, and*
> *all humankind! Brilliant as the sun and moon!*

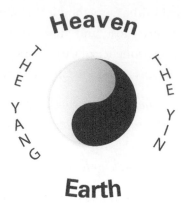

The Breaths of Yin and Yang, the Way of the Elixir

The Three Powers are Heaven as one, earth as two and man as three: the three add together both the one and the two. Thus does the human frame combine and bring together both Heaven and earth.

> *NOTE: This is a central tenet of Daoism: the microcosm of the human form and the macrocosm of Heaven and earth are one and the same process. Each man and woman is just a small Heaven.*

THE *WESTERN MOUNTAIN RECORDS* STATE THAT IN ancient times Hua Tuo displayed the Five-Animal Play and created the art of 'inducting the breath' (*daoyin*). He saw that people lived their lives in idleness and stagnancy – therefore he taught them to bend and awaken their physical bodies; he caused their lives also to awaken and to become vigorous.

Later folks followed him and called this 'circulating the breath round and round', and searched for a further result – but this was the wrong way to go about it!

In ancient times Zhen Yi met a certain woman on the Path, and for a long time went hungry, studying the breathing methods of the hibernating tortoise. Thus he acquired life and ended his years without dying a natural death.

Later folks followed him and called this simply 'living on the breath', and searched for the Medicinal Elixir by this Path, but this was the wrong way to go about it!

Another adept looked closely at how eating certain foods throws the juices of the people into disorder, one organ being loved and another hated, one kind of breath being strengthened and another weakened. So then, by omitting certain of these foodstuffs, he simplified and blended them into the organ-breaths.

Later folks followed him and called this using 'body rations', but this was the wrong way to go about it!

A certain Liudong proposed the law: if the True Yin and Yang were in excess, then to 'guide the child', and if insufficient, then to 'kill the devil', strengthening and weakening where each was fitting; and later generations followed him by clutching at the 'glory of the sun' and 'bright light of the moon'. This was carried out in order to acquire the proper breath of Heaven and earth, but this was the wrong way to go about it!

And also in ancient times Master Guang Zheng taught the Yellow Emperor the arts of the bedchamber lest he should lose or mislay the True Breath.

He spoke of the 'path of fostering and sustaining', and on how to properly conquer a foe. But he did not discuss accurately and make explicit sexual matters, the 'clutching battle of man and woman', but only how to rob the breath of a woman to foster his own.

Later folks followed him, calling this 'one person building another'; they 'clutched at the breath' and 'returned the seed' but only harmed others and injured themselves. They were hoping for long life, but this was entirely the wrong way to go about it.

NOTE: This is mentioned in the Daoist Zhuangzi classic.

It was Master Guang Zheng who instructed the Yellow Emperor in the many paths of 'fostering and sustaining' – and for a long time he did not see any results. But at Emei Mountain, taking 'internal affairs' as his model, he managed to develop an 'external elixir' and rebuild a long-standing weakness to compensate for the harm of accumulated injuries.

Later folks followed him, but used passionless stones and minerals, forging and smelting in the smoke and grime, dissecting up the foetus to see if it contained a treasure, perhaps seeking to ascend above into Heaven, perhaps to evade death and lengthen their lives. But this was entirely the wrong way to go about it!

> *NOTE: I visited this historic site in modern*
> *Sichuan province in 1986.*

Bian Que, the doctor, commenting on the *Lingshu* medical classic, spoke of using the nose to guide in the clean breath, the mouth expelling the polluted breath, and then retaining it slightly and doing this for twenty-four breaths, to make one ounce of Fire.

He then smelted out the True Lead like a 'dancing yellow shoot', and called this a 'Yang Foetus', smelting out the True Mercury like an 'enclosed lotus bud', calling this a 'Yin Foetus'. Once the Foetus existed, the breath departed; the breath departed and the spirit was retained.

Thus he said it was possible to 'retain this physical body and depart this world', and over a period of time to 'enter the company of Sages and transcend earthly matters'.

Later folks followed this technique by 'taking in more and letting out less', wishing to gather in the breath in order to form a foetus. They retained the breath and this became their method. But this was quite the wrong way to go about it!

The *Nine Immortals* classic spoke of 'using fire when the disease is great' and 'using water when the disease is slight'.

When you use fire, you take in the breath, returning it throughout the whole body. The True Breath passes throughout the four limbs, and the Yin Devils and Spirits observe it and dare not come near.

When you use water, you take in the breath, again returning it throughout the whole body; and it becomes like water, a bubbling spring, a fountain established within. So then the mind can travel to the place where the disease exists, the breath and blood flowing on progressively, on their own account, without any blockages or interruptions.

Later folks followed this technique and sat alone retaining the breath; using the tongue 'to the left rotating, to the right returning', drawing back in the precious saliva, gargling with it and swallowing it, returning it on to the stomach, and transmitting it back out to penetrate the body. This they called 'rinsing and washing' and thereby grew a Yellow Sprout, desiring to create a Great Medicine. But this was the wrong way to go about it!

The classic on *Penetrating the Mysteries* spoke on 'guarding the Path of non-action and acquiring the principle of natural behaviour', of 'becoming clear and unblinkered, quiet and delaying moving', of 'shifting the spirit to the wilderness of rarity' and of 'safeguarding the body on the path of kindness and longevity'.

Then, as no single thought arose, all anxieties ceased, and they lengthened their lives and 'preserved their years'; they were peaceful and at ease, happy and content.

Later folks followed this path, without understanding really how to 'choose quiet and cut off all traces', to be perfectly silent and forget all workings. Thus all their lives they were not aware of the possibility of any further results. This was the wrong way to go about it!

The Inner View of the Treasure classic says, 'Do not let the outer world enter in, do not let the inner world seep out.' Then, with the spirit and understanding naturally guarded, you are to close the eyes and view within, lowering the ruling Fire to the lower belly, in order to disperse yellow clouds along the Four Limbs so it spreads out, coming and going, quite naturally within the 'old pot' of the body.

Later folks followed this technique, their bodies like dried wood, their hearts like dead ashes; diligently they guarded the Void, lost in dark silence, the Yin spirit exiting the Heavenly Gate, thus to 'slip foetal rebirth'. But this was entirely the wrong way to go about it!

Then there are also methods like stretching out the neck as a tortoise, and so on. These methods derive from the mountains and are said to enable you to understand your own nature. The inner fire is used to smelt and catch hold of your seed – in fact, to sustain your life. But these are not merely of no benefit; they actually do harm.

These later folks who practised methods such as these actually possessed a little understanding but lacked any true knowledge. They themselves gave birth to the lesser methods and schools. They all linked together, supporting and reinforcing each other, misleading and encouraging doubt amongst the later generations, until day after day they caused the Great Path to be swept up and lost.

They never knew how to 'look up in respect' to the heavens or 'bow down in respect' to the earth – or to join silently in fit accord with the rise and fall of all things, and to display the general rule of Yin and Yang, the coming and going of the sun and moon, the Hun and Po-souls.

> NOTE: *The key here is to 'join silently in accord with the rise and fall of all things'. To display the general rule of Yin and Yang, the coming and going of the sun and moon, the Hun and Po-souls will finally enable you to attain your goal; in other words, to act gently and naturally. The description Shi Jianwu gives below shows the correct attitude. All the methods listed above fall short of the mark.*

When the single breath begins to first surface, it appears as the Yin and Yang of the single self; once the Five Cycles are split up, they create the water and fire of the single self; yet within the fire lies water, whilst within the water lies fire.

Within the fire lies 'a tangled confusion', and is borne the Yin (water), its substance being the *water of the True One*.

At the same time, within the water 'darkly occurring' is carried the Yang (fire), its essence being the *vapour of the Proper Yang*.

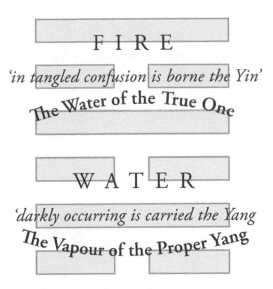

Married together to form a Medicine

Both breaths married together will be able to form an inner Medicine. Then, once this is sustained, it turns into a Golden Elixir – and then it is possible to become a land-based Immortal!

> *NOTE: This important last section is the defining moment, a description of the knowledge in these records. It begins with elemental cosmology: heaven, earth and man, water (cooling) and fire (heating). Later the impetus turns to the idea of life, as in the human foetus in the womb – water and fire joined together 'in tangled confusion', 'darkly occurring' – this identifies the mystery of life;[1] and then, to the later work of the adept, taking the Yin from the Yang and the Yang from the Yin, leading to the marriage of the True Yin and True Yang. Being 'true' signifies our 'before-Heaven' or 'before-we-are-born' existence. As these two, the True Yin and True Yang, marry together, in*

---

1   These important phrases (from the *Tao-te Ching*, Ch.21) occur again in Chapter 5, 'Knowing the Materials'.

doing so they form the Elixir. Their existence thus consists
of 'closeness with no disrespect'. Here I am speaking
from experience, not mere thought or theory. Later we
will see how to rise above and 'walk in the divine'.

3

Knowing the Individual

The true method involves nothing else than being at peace within, and not labouring at the work; and if you labour, then not to toil…in order to preserve intact the soft line of the passage of the breath…

THE GREAT PATH IS UNLIKE ANYTHING ELSE – ALTHOUGH full of virtue, it appears as if absent; its light shaded, its traces few, its track unclear, protecting the reality of its position, that people may pass by unknowingly and unheeding.

If the Great Path is not secured within your own person, your words will be scorned by others; and if its business does not fully occupy your thoughts, although you speak of the Path and put on airs, you will only seek to dominate people, and they will eventually pass you by.

For the fellow who makes a study of this truth, a knowledge of how to deal with people is an essential prerequisite. When acquiring companions, listen to how they speak and watch how they behave; when looking for a method, scrutinise its main principles and judge by results.

Neither exploit others nor neglect what they say. Guard against disputes carefully. Do not use your speech to influence or try to influence them; protect against perfecting a particular style. Pure knowledge always contains small irregularities – for we all start off ignorant to end up a sage!

The fellow who makes a study of this truth holds up a mirror to himself, by which he may know others. But he really only knows himself. This is to emphatically promote the Noble and Peerless Path!

> *NOTE: An emphasis on being certain, and true self-knowledge. But knowledge of others is also a prerequisite. The text advises care in choosing companions. Do not try to perfect a particular style. Through gaining knowledge of others, you get to know yourself; through reflecting upon yourself and accepting your own failings, you may acquire a knowledge of others.*

THROUGHOUT ALL TIMES, THE SAINTS AND SAGES OF Old, although they combined together the wisdom of all men and sages, and shone with the utmost brilliance, they never committed to study unless they had first sought out a teacher. This is stated in the *Western Mountain Records*.

This implies that to devote yourself to knowledge is not nearly as good as to devote yourself to a teacher. The teacher yields the pattern for the pupil.

> *NOTE: A clear message. Oral transmission is the essential prerequisite for learning this method.*

The Yellow Emperor sought out a Master from the Red Pines, and after six months acquired the *Book of Internal Prohibitions*, succeeding in protecting against his outer loss.

Liu-An 'Jade' taught Wang Dao 'Source' all his life's small arts and methods, but he never spoke of any affair to do with the secret of 'fostering and sustaining', whilst Zhu spent time with Mr Hu and to the end of time they could not be separated.

Fang-Tan came across the Golden Flower and followed it far and near. Qian-San came across the 'Watery Toad' and thenceforth gained the Method of the Three Vehicles. He released his will bit by bit, and the Yang came to him; he exhausted the teachings of the Nine Firings, and all was complete. Mr Wang had experience of many methods of long-life practice and thereby prolonged his years until they came close to those of a Great Immortal. Then, whilst chattering and laughing aimlessly to others, he disclosed the Great Path.

Man Fu met True Master 'Deep Cavern' on the highway and, whilst he ran next to him, immediately ended any doubts he had concerning the workings of nature.

Through all ten thousand generations there has never been a lack of Holy Immortals willing to help ferry you across to the Southern Isles. But if you do not come across a fellow who makes a study of the truth, all talk will come to nothing.

> *NOTE: The true method is quite easily found. All that is needed is devotion to a proper teacher. The prerequisite for 'knowing' is that there is one who 'knows'. All the above are historical examples of this.*

But some folks seem to have an appearance of being 'in the Dao', dressed in ancient-looking garb. They argue and talk glibly, describing how you can 'touch a Holy Immortal', although at all times they are committing crimes of the commonplace. They may have studied the matter but they have never encountered it. These are the *first* category of people.

Others take the matter very seriously, but without much joy in their lives. They have no faith in the workings of Heaven: they make light of their daily routine and place more importance on impressing other people and possessions. They casually befriend men who are twisted and evil, not those of a happy disposition.

Although they are happy to meet others, they do not listen to what they say; and if they hear them, they do not take in what is being said. In the end they achieve nothing as the mortal and immortal world are set at odds with each other.

This category of people may have encountered the matter but have never really touched upon it. They are the *second* category.

Then there are those of extensive intellect and unswerving devotion, who ply you with problems and close-argued questions, but even if they touch upon the true answer, they prove to be idle. They are happy one moment and then depressed the next; in the morning they say one thing but by the evening they have changed their mind. They sit in meditation a short while and then expect immediate enlightenment. They may have touched upon the matter but have not retained it. These are the *third* category of people.

In addition all these folk make long speeches, devise wild practices, and search out strange theories, 'throwing away the opportunity of the moment and squandering the day'. How can they ever get a result!

> *NOTE: Three categories of people who miss out on the Path. They are those who have studied the matter, but never encountered it; those who have encountered the matter, but never touched upon it; and those who have touched the matter, but never retained it.*

The highest category of people amongst the Ancients first made an extensive study of the alchemical literature; next they committed themselves entirely to a companion on the Path. They took the Great Path as their total topic of conversation, thereby committing themselves without entertaining any strange theories – joining all mankind on the Path, and thereby teaching without wild or disreputable practices.

But alas! The world is stupid and people can only think of themselves. Not one can separate wisdom from foolishness. They cheapen themselves in their work, without distinguishing right and wrong. If you discuss this knowledge with those who are already lost, you will never convince them.

Throughout all the ages, the seekers of truth amongst the highest Sages, before they fostered 'refining' themselves into an Immortal, fostered the 'sustaining' of the body, mind and spirit.

Now people say such things as 'washing and bathing, you should avoid the wind'. And they also say:

> Find a quiet room within a silent building,
> Close the eyes and dim the heart.
> Stretch out the body, sitting upright,
> To enable the 'originating breath' to rise upwards –
> Then it encircles fully the four limbs,
> Reaching upwards into the brain.

This is the 'true method of cleansing the Elixir', but it is also a million miles away from 'the dialogue of water and fire'.

They also speak of not spitting far as it injures the breath, not walking fast as it injures the tendons, not straining the eyes as it dims their sparkle, not straining the ears as it injures the kidneys, not standing all day as it wounds the bones, and not lying all day as it wounds the muscles.

They say that too much sleep clouds the mind, rapid drinking dissipates the spark of life, too much sweating injures the blood and too much exertion exhausts and wounds the body. They think that speeding carts and racing horses confuse the person and shock the mind; and that gazing at lofty structures and ascending to perilous heights will scatter the Po-soul and disperse the Hun.

But the true method of sustaining the body involves nothing else than being at peace within, without labouring at the work – and if you do labour, then not to toil.

It involves remaining still within and not flinching – but if you do flinch, then not to worry.

> Refill yourself without,
> Bank up yourself within.

Then you may contemplate the Five Cycles of Form, earth, fire, water, wood and metal, which preserve intact the soft line of the breath.

That is all there is to it. Be firm without and true within – for then, when both these predominate, you may be preserved for an eternity.

4

為

Knowing the Timing

Do not confuse the hour! Settle the moment and you secure your destiny. How could you then be far from the Path?

THESE PEOPLE AND THINGS WHO POSSESS A PHYSICAL form cannot lack a name, but then if they have a name, their destiny is somewhat difficult to foretell. This is a statement from the book on *Opening up the Mysteries*. This book continues: their majesty is modelled on Heaven and earth, Yin and Yang, rising and falling without losing place; their brilliance modelled on the sun and moon, their souls on the Hun and Po, coming and going at their own pace.

But a single hair's breadth out and this process of constant inversion is lost. If Yin and Yang come adrift, the succession of the seasons turns into chaos and then they can no longer bring about the birth, correct development and completion of the ten thousand creatures; if the climate of cold and heat misses its turn, the seasons are disrupted and all nature can no longer circulate about the single breath of life.

*NOTE: This single chapter further describes how the
Sages of Old took after the ways of nature themselves,
to 'join silently in fit accord with the rise and fall of all
things, displaying the general rule of Yin and Yang, the*

coming and going of the sun and moon, the Hun and Po-
souls.' The business of 'having a name' or 'lacking a name'
derives from the Tao-te Ching (Ch.1), where it states:
nameless is the beginning of Heaven and earth. The image
of modelling ourselves on Heaven and earth, Yin and
Yang, and the sun and moon permeates the Neijing and
Yijing, two of the oldest texts in the Chinese canon.

Man is the most precious of creatures, the spiritual haven of the single breath of life.

Suppose that, in his majesty, he took Heaven and earth as his image, he could then not possibly subvert his rightful place in their rise and fall; suppose that, in his brilliance, he took the sun and moon as his model, he could then not possibly fall out of step with the pace of their rule.

Settle the moment, and you secure your destiny. How could you then be far from the Path?

NOTE: This is the crux – for the human form to
take on the majesty of Heaven and earth, to adopt
the brilliance of the sun and moon, and to invert Yin
and Yang within. Thereby, through aping the heavens
you may become one with them. Macrocosm and
microcosm reflect each other, the one and the same.

THE GREAT PATH HAS NO PHYSICAL FORM YET IT BRINGS into being and is able to sustain all Heaven and earth, warmth and coolness – whilst cold and heat join and cross over in a single year. They join and cross over without missing a single step and one year follows on another, and then another. This idea comes from the *Western Mountain Records*.

The Great Path shows no emotion yet it drives around the sun and moon: first quarter, full moon, last quarter and new moon, they come and go in a single month, coming and going without missing a moment, and one month follows on another, and then another.

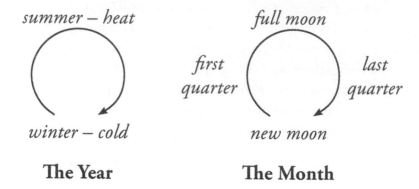

The Year   **The Month**

The Great Path has no name, yet it sustains and helps develop all the ten thousand things. However, this does not mean simply that in spring they are born and in summer they flourish, because the elm drops its seeds in the spring; and it does not mean simply that they are harvested in autumn and stored in winter, because other plants act contrary to this.

All creatures follow the timing of season and day to receive the breath, and then follow the breath to send out life, without knowing that like plants and trees they should act like this.

But the most magical of them all is man. If this does not dawn upon him – and he sustains the reality of his own nature, and fosters his actual torso and body, how can he do anything!

> *NOTE: This is to display the naturalness of*
> *humankind. We simply form one body with all*
> *natural forces. It is imperative we understand this*
> *fact and work to sustain our own True nature.*

The crane knows half the night, the swallow understands only the summer, finding their cause in Yin and being affected by Yang, following on their natural conditions. Water washes away soil, the snake at the close of the day does not cross a rocky path, and in spring months of its own accord leaves the valley. Thus without knowing how or why they do so, animals, birds and beasts all act in such ways.

But since the most honourable of them all is man, how could he then not also yield to the time? How can he avoid sustaining the Primal Yang and withdrawing and storing the True Breath, how indeed?

NOTE: Again, all living things are following nature.

If we do not know this, then our breath is lost and scattered, and eight hundred and ten feet of originating breath, over a single day, will be harmed. Do you not yet understand that the True Breath and its Great Circulation follows the cycle of the skies: in spring resting in the liver, in summer resting in the heart, in autumn resting in the lungs, in winter resting in the kidneys?

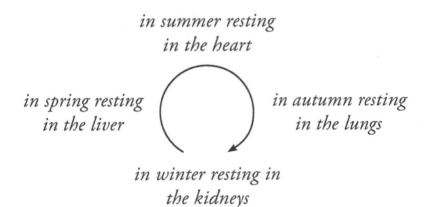

in summer resting
in the heart

in spring resting   *in autumn resting*
in the liver   *in the lungs*

in winter resting in
the kidneys

The True Breath and its Great Circulation

Whilst the originating breath and its small circulation around the body follows the day and the sun: at midnight resting in the kidneys, at dawn resting in the liver, at midday resting in the heart, at dusk resting in the lungs.

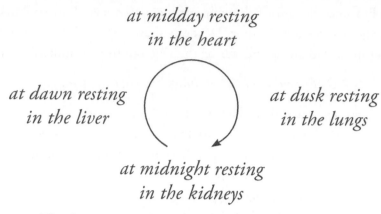

*at midday resting
in the heart*

*at dawn resting
in the liver*

*at dusk resting
in the lungs*

*at midnight resting
in the kidneys*

The Originating Breath and its Small Circulation

Heaven and earth contain spring, summer, autumn and winter; the sun and moon display first quarter, full moon, last quarter and new moon; the human form experiences midnight, midday, dusk and dawn. In just accord they all lie at their proper post, united together.

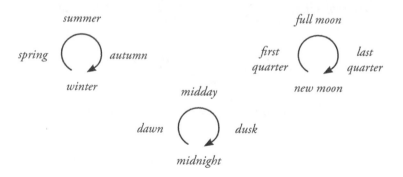

Winter represents the Yin; within the Yin is born the Yang as warmth, so then we have spring. This is Yang being host and Yin being the guest. Within the Yang is born the Yang again as heat, so then we have summer; summer represents the Yang. Within the Yang is born the Yin as a coolness, so then we have autumn. This is Yin being host and Yang being the guest. Within the Yin is born the Yin again, as coldness, so then we have winter; winter represents the Yin. This describes the four seasons of Heaven and earth.

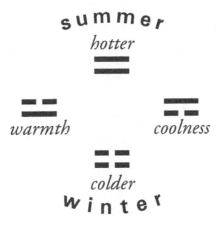

The new moon arrives, and it is all dark. Then within the Po-soul is born the Hun as light, and we have the first quarter. After the first quarter the Hun is the body whilst the Po is the function. Within the Hun is again born the Hun, and this is called 'full moon'. It is full moon, so all is light. Then within the Hun-soul is born the Po as darkness, so then we have the last quarter. After the last quarter the Po is the body whilst the Hun is the function. Within the Po is again born the Po, and this is called 'new moon'. This describes the four seasons of the sun and moon.

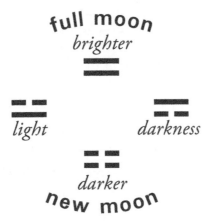

Heaven and earth comprise three hundred and sixty days; the sun and moon comprise three hundred and sixty hours (360 hours = 15 days, half a month); man contains three hundred and sixty measured joints.

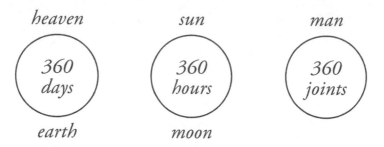

Heaven and earth comprise twenty-four breaths (2 x 12 months); the sun and moon have twenty-four measures throughout the year (24 fortnights); man partakes of twenty-four hours.

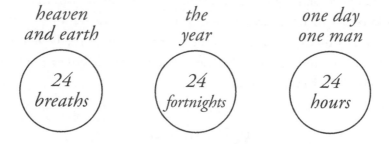

From the hours of midnight until the time of midday the breath is living and Yang; from the hours of midday until the time of midnight the breath is dying and Yin. Early dawn, early morn, midday, afternoon, midnight and early evening are the six periods the Yang is being born; dawn, just before midday, just after midday, dusk, just before midnight and just after midnight are the six periods the Yin is being born.

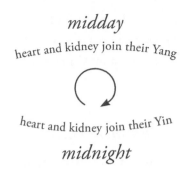

midday

heart and kidney join their Yang

heart and kidney join their Yin

midnight

At midday the kidney-breath joins with the heart-breath, above and below, and it is the moment the Yang energies coalesce; at midnight the heart-breath joins with the kidney-breath, below and above, and it is the moment the Yin energies coalesce.

midday

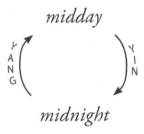

midnight

The Hun-soul is the Yang within the Yin, its breath is born at the very first glimpse of dawn; the Po-soul is the Yin without the Yang, its breath is born as dusk draws to a close.

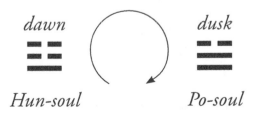

dawn   *dusk*

Hun-soul   *Po-soul*

However sustaining the Yang does not simply depend upon spring and summer. If you sustain the Yang simply during spring and summer, the breath merely exists in the heart and liver. And sustaining the Yin does not simply depend upon autumn and winter. If you sustain the Yin simply during autumn and winter, the breath merely exists in the lungs and kidney.

summer – heart

Yin and Yang sustained throughout

liver – spring   *lungs – autumn*

winter – kidneys

NOTE: You cannot just simply copy Yin and Yang in nature. You must discover and sustain the True Yin and True Yang.

Just after midsummer the True Mercury builds up within the Purple Palace within the heart; just after midwinter, the True Lead builds up within the Cinnabar Field or belly.

just after midsummer the
True Mercury builds

just after midwinter the
True Lead builds

As the Wood cycle crosses with the twenty-five measures of the Heavenly Cycle, it is the time for the trigram Sun, the gentle wind of the spring; so as Yang crosses Yang, at that moment, withdraw it to form the Great Medicine. As the Metal cycle joins with the twenty-five measures of the Spiritual Token, it is the time for the trigram Qian, the stern father of autumn; so as Yin crosses Yin, at that moment, smelt it and name it the Elixir of Return.

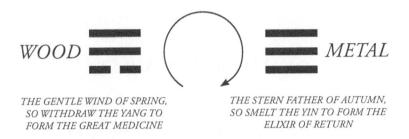

WOOD

THE GENTLE WIND OF SPRING,
SO WITHDRAW THE YANG TO
FORM THE GREAT MEDICINE

METAL

THE STERN FATHER OF AUTUMN,
SO SMELT THE YIN TO FORM THE
ELIXIR OF RETURN

Smelt the physical body and raise a fire, making certain this comes about before the breath rises; gather in the fire and return it to the dark, making sure this makes use of the opportunity of the Yin descending.

TAKING TIME AS PRIORITY
to smelt the breath, employ the
climates of the three cinnabar
fields so 'the Yin returns'

to smelt the physical body, use
the chances given by the five
cycles 'of mutual self-control'
TAKING BREATH AS PRIORITY

As you smelt the physical body, you depart from this dusty world, taking the breath as priority and using the chances given to you by the Five Cycles' system of mutual self-control; then, as you smelt the breath, you transcend earthly matters, taking the timing of material objects as priority and employing the climates of the Three Cinnabar Fields wherein the Yin returns.

> If the Fellow who makes a study of this Truth
> Does not see results, it is because –
> His breath flourishes but he does not withdraw it,
> When damaged he does not repair it,
> When scattered he does not regroup it,
> When he joins with it he cannot employ it,
> When absent he does not inquire after it,
> And finally when it does return he cannot smelt it.

He is ignorant of the moment of Yin and Yang 'joining and crossing', and lacks any method whereby he can capture them. He 'confuses the hour, is mistaken on the day', and is not aware of any graduations in his work.

DAMAGED (REPAIR IT)

FLOURISHES (WITHDRAW IT)   RETURNS (SMELT IT)

ABSENT (ENQUIRE AFTER IT)
JOIN WITH IT (EMPLOY IT)
SCATTERED (REGROUP IT)

Taking the Breath as Priority

How then can he compare his longevity to that of Heaven and earth or stand as solid as the sun and moon!

NOTE: The first part of the book on the Knowledge introduces the Path, Method, Individual, Timing and Materials. This chapter on the Timing reveals its true substance.

5

物

Knowing the Materials

Take the materials to investigate the matter in hand
and the Yang is comparable to movement, whilst the
Yin stands for quietness...but these matters can be
over-discussed...

THE ANNALS RECORDED ON THE VAULT OF THE SKY RELATE
how if you use spoken words to describe the Way, you only uncover
a few shreds and remnants – because to find the Way you have to
forget about the words; and if you use visual images to search out its
meaning, you find only a slight semblance of things – because to find
its meaning, you have to forget all about the visual images.

Nevertheless, the Way dwells in words, by means of the former
knowledge informing the latter. It is not that the words are totally
insufficient because you search, through them, for the principle. In
addition, it is also true that the meaning of the Way rests in images,
as it is a greater enlightenment that bursts through a lesser. It is not
that the images are totally inadequate – as you make a plea, through
them, for the reality.

Words reveal principle, just as images display reality. So what can
we say? That the Great Way stands shrouded in meaning, in a place
of secret understanding, beyond all images and words.

At the beginning, we use detailed speech and convoluted expressions, fearful lest someone misunderstand us; we compare different materials and employ images, fearful lest someone may go uninformed. Then eventually our aim is achieved, the Way is retained, and its method does not rest in spoken words; the mind is one, the meaning clear, and its significance not resting in images.

> *NOTE: This chapter on the materials is the most detailed so far. At the beginning we are reminded that words and images are only partially successful in telling us of reality. That is why the Great Method is shrouded in meaning. Names and shapes should not be taken too seriously.*

THE *WESTERN MOUNTAIN RECORDS* STATE THAT THAT which lies beyond our sight is the Path, and that that which lies within our sight is the 'utensil'. The unseen takes the seen as its foundation, whilst the Path picks up a utensil because it finds it useful.

This is just as the *Secret Book of Zhongli* says:

Take the heart as heaven,
The kidneys as the earth,
The lungs as the moon,
And the liver as the sun.

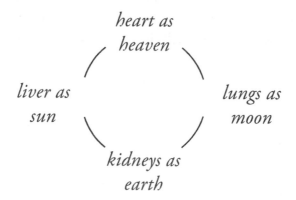

The sun and moon, Heaven and earth are materials of great brilliance.

The True Strange Sayings of Dark Cui state:

> Consider the kidney breath to be as a little child
> And the heart's fluid becomes a mild maiden.
> The liver breath the Yang within the Yin,
> The Hun-soul within the sun;
> The lung breath the Yin within the Yang,
> The Po-soul within the moon.

Here the child, the maiden and Hun and Po-souls are fashioned materials that possess great magic and are deeply spiritual.

In a similar fashion, four pictorial images occur: the heart as a 'red bird', the kidneys as 'dark warriors', the liver as a 'green dragon' and the lungs as a 'white tiger'.

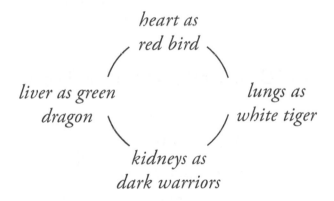

Lord Ge Immortal states: The little child is the vapour of the Proper Yang within the heart's fluid. The mild maiden is the water of the True One within the kidney-breath. The golden Duke is the Old Yang of the lungs. The yellow Dame is the Yang when still small and weak, so then convey her back to the 'lower field' (*dantian*). She has sufficient fluid to make up the Old Yin. When the kidney fluid reaches the spleen fluid, the True Yang comes close to the Young Yin — so although the Yin is feeble and weak, it is just there at the right time to convey it back to the 'lower field' (*dantian*). Here you have a complete and detailed description of the Four Images!

The True Fellow 'Supreme Purity' states: Once the Art of the Five Cycles is crafted topsy-turvy, the Dragon comes out from the fire; whilst if the Five Cycles are not actively loosened, the Tiger is born from the water.

> *NOTE: The Dragon (wood), originally from the East, comes out from the fire in the south; the Tiger (metal), actually belonging to the West, is born from the water in the north. This most famous rhyme by the poet Li Bai 'Supreme Purity' is quoted again in Chapter 17. These animals are crafted topsy-turvy, born from out the water and fire.*

The Dragon, originally a creature of the Eastern direction of Jia-Yi, yet comes out from the fire; he arrives within the heart's fluid as the vapour of the Proper Yang. So then this is called 'the Yang Dragon emerging from the Palace of the Trigram Li-fire'.

The Dragon comes

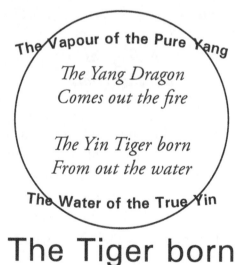

The Vapour of the Pure Yang

The Yang Dragon
Comes out the fire

The Yin Tiger born
From out the water

The Water of the True Yin

The Tiger born

The Animals crafted Topsy-turvy

The Tiger, actually a creature of the Western direction of Geng-Xin, is yet born from the water; she lies within the kidneys' vapour as the water of the True One. So then she is called 'the Yin Tiger born at the Post of the Trigram Kan-water'.

Nevertheless, the Dragon is a Yang creature and to rise up aloft is what he does best; he exists within water as the Yang within the Yin. Thus he may be matched with the heart's fluid, as the vapour of the Proper Yang.

The Tiger is a Yin creature and to wrestle to the ground is what she does best; she dwells on the earth as the Yin within the Yang. Thus she may be matched with the vapour of the kidneys, as the water of the True One.

Lao Zi says, 'in tangled confusion, yet within it lies a substance': this is because within the kidneys' vapour there is also a fluid. It is, in fact, bearing the Yin. He also says, 'darkly occurring, yet within it lies an essence': this is because within the heart's fluid, there is actually a vapour. It is, in fact, carrying the Yang.

> NOTE: These two expressions are also explained in
> Chapter 2 on The Method. The Tao-te Ching collection
> (Ch.21) states: 'in tangled confusion, yet within it lies some
> substance…darkly occurring, yet within it lies vitality.'
> These two phrases partly refer to the Yang substance lying
> within the heart-Yin fluid and the Yin essence lying within
> the kidney-Yang vapour. Jia-Yi and Geng-Xin relate to
> rising and falling, dawn and dusk, opening and close.

Our True Lord Yin states: The Proper Breath of the Northern Regions is spoken of as the 'Chain-and-Bucket River Pump'. The 'chain-and-bucket' refers to the transportation of materials up from water to dry land; the chain with its buckets arrives and departs tirelessly, carrying up water, thus it is known as the River Pump.

This gains a meaning within the human body, as amongst the myriad Yin in the lower body there occurs a single speck of originating Yang ascending up, steaming above to give birth to the originating breath.

The kidney-breath transmits to the liver-breath, the liver-breath transmits to the heart-breath, the heart-breath transmits to the lung-breath, and the lung-breath transmits to the kidney-breath.

This is called the Lesser Chain-and-Bucket River Pump...'and at your elbow the Gold is shown in splendour'.

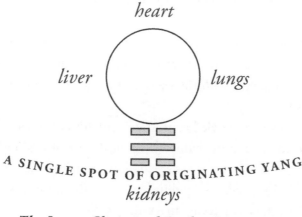

The Lesser Chain-and-Bucket River Pump

Then, from the tailbone point it begins to move – from the Lower Pass it crosses over the Central Pass and from the Central Pass to the Upper Pass, from the Upper Pass reaching the Central Field, and from the Central Field reaching the Lower Field. This is called the Greater Chain-and-Bucket River Pump.

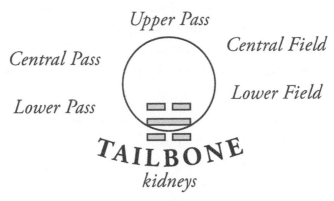

The Greater Chain-and-Bucket River Pump

As the Pure Yin falls beneath, the true fire of its own accord arrives; and as the Pure Yang rises above, the true fire of its own accord begins. The one rising, the one sinking, both seen together in front of the Twelve-Tiered Pagoda;[1] drop by drop the Elixir of Return is born, then bringing into existence the Golden Shining Ten Thousand Times Mighty Path. So then this is called the Imperial Greater Chain-and-Bucket River Pump.

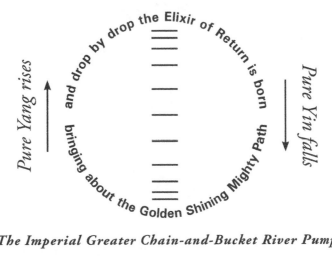

The Imperial Greater Chain-and-Bucket River Pump

---

1   Thoracic spine.

The chain-and-bucket transports the water of the river, just as the breath moves and exists within the blood sub-vessels; and within this breath is hidden the true water, just like a chain and its buckets having something carried within. This is a detailed description of the Chain-and-Bucket River Pump.

> *NOTE: The three Chain-and-Bucket River Pumps explain*
> *the movement of the breath within the blood. Within the*
> *breath is hidden the true water, carried about, through*
> *and through the body, by the 'chain and buckets'.*

Master Guang Zheng used these 'internal affairs' to educate the Yellow Emperor, but after a long time there were still no visible results, until on Emei Mountain he developed the idea of speaking of a Great Medicine.

Within the Five Metals, Lead represents all black metals, and from these black metals you then select Silver; within the Eight Minerals, Sand represents all red minerals, and from these red minerals you then select Mercury.

SAND

select Mercury from within

|

select Silver from within

LEAD

You take the Mercury and Silver to form a Jewelled Substance; this is why we talk about Lead and Mercury.

The Lead represents the loins within which the True Breath is stored; the Mercury represents Yin and Yang joined together in the single self as the true seed-essences.

MERCURY

Yin and Yang joined
in true seed-essences

|

LEAD

the True Breath
stored in the loins

The True Yin and True Yang are that which form the Great Medicine – given the 'timing of the firing', they may proceed without interruption; and as their true seed-essences are transformed into Mercury, Mercury is transformed into Sand, and the Sand into an Elixir. This describes what happens to the True Lead.

Gold, 'splendid in an instant, vapourising', enters into the Upper Palace, from the crown then entering into the Lower Field – and the true fire is born in front, rising up to enter into the Muddy Pill, from the heart crossing over to the Double Tower, one Yin and one Yang, water above and fire beneath, creating a situation which is 'already complete' (Hexagram 63). As this progresses on to the Primal Sea,[2] it is known as the Imperial Golden Elixir. This describes what happens to the True Mercury. This is just how it goes.

---

2   Lower belly.

The above supplies a picture of the workings of the Lead and Mercury in detail.

Now take these materials to investigate the matter in hand and the Yang is comparable to movement and rising up, whilst the Yin stands for quietness and consolidation. Yet these materials can be over-discussed, and their images over-relied upon – just stay with the two energies of the Pure Yin and Pure Yang that coalesce together into the Great Medicine.

And yet also there is the True Yin within the Yang and the True Yang within the Yin; namely, the Yang intersecting the Yin, the Yin intersecting the Yang, the Yang intersecting the Yang, and the Yin intersecting the Yin, a fourfold intersection of Yin and Yang. Second, there is the Yin joining the Yang, the Yang joining the Yin, the Yin joining the Yin, and the Yang joining the Yang, again, a fourfold joining of Yin and Yang.

In all its majesty, this fourfold 'intersection and junction' corresponds to the eight divisions of Heaven and earth, and in all their brilliance, to the eight territories of the sun and moon.

YANG
The True Yin within

Yang intersecting Yin, Yin intersecting Yang
Yang intersecting Yang, Yin intersecting Yin

Yin joining the Yang, Yang joining the Yin
Yin joining the Yin, Yang joining the Yang

The True Yang within
YIN

The True Yin and Yang

But too much rendering and over-discussion not only hampers the mind and injures the breath, but also makes for differences between things.

Choose to 'neglect the hour, mistake the day' and in the end there will never be any real benefit!

The Sustaining

6

生

Sustaining Life

> Knowing to be alive to the sustaining of the breath ensures it does not fail...so then quieten the mind and still the thoughts, close the eyes and straighten up the body...

PEOPLE AND CREATURES DIFFER IN SHAPE, BUT IN receiving life they are all the same. The *True Book on the Three Primals* states the following:

The breath and the Hun-soul is acquired from the heavens; the body and Po-soul from the earth. When there is as yet no form, and no image, we arrive from 'out of a void', as our own father's seed and mother's blood; thus from out of nothing there emerges something. After three hundred days the foetus is complete, and when the foetus is complete and the breath ready, we are born; thus from out of nothing there emerges something.

But if we are not skilled at sustaining this life, then from something we return back to nothing. This is just how it is.

NOTE: This means premature death. Below
we will see how we may sustain life.

As the blood and breath are strong, spirit and breath come into being, which may then give birth to a little child; once the blood and breath decline, they result in the Hun and Po-souls returning them back to the heavens and earth.

> Within life is born a Chaos;
> From Chaos we may halt at life;
> When our breaths are broken or the spirit gone,
> There is no longer any chance for life.
> This is just how it is.

The best of men and rulers always set their hearts on capturing life, but not knowing the moment or method, they took as their model the heavens and earth, and as their thumb-line the Sun and Moon.

> Once the Yin is exhausted the Yang is born,
> Once the Yang is exhausted the Yin is born,
> Life follows upon life unfailing –
> In such a fashion Heaven and earth endure;
> The Po departs and the Hun arrives,
> The Hun departs and the Po arrives,
> Coming and going unceasing –
> So do the sun and moon endure.

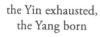
the Yin exhausted,
the Yang born

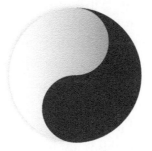

the Yang exhausted,
the Yin born

It is knowing to be alive to sustaining the breath that ensures it does not fail, and being alive to sustaining the body that means it does not ail; never missing out on sustaining them both, within and without, enables us to acquire our true identity along with our enduring partners, Heaven and earth, the sun and moon.

> *NOTE: The task is simple – to ape the heavens in pursuit of their enduring strength, and to follow the earth in search of its bountiful support. Then we may indeed sustain human life.*

THE *WESTERN MOUNTAIN RECORDS* STATE THAT through countless ages, the saints and sages have all spoken of the method of sustaining life, and recorded its many theories. This has happened countless times.

Again they have spoken of 'reducing selfishness and curbing desire'; reducing selfishness and curbing desire will sustain the heart.

Again they have spoken of 'ceasing all thought and forgetting skill'; ceasing all thought and forgetting skill will sustain the spirit.

Again they have spoken of 'regulating our diet'; regulating our diet will sustain the physical body.

Again they have spoken of 'regulating business and leisure'; regulating business and leisure will sustain the blood.

Again they have spoken of 'taking in the pure and discharging the impure'; taking in the pure and discharging the impure will sustain the breath.

Again they have spoken of 'ending licentious activities and guarding against sexual desire'; ending licentious activities and guarding against sexual desire will sustain the fluid-essences.

But the Way of sustaining life is not based upon any of these activities. Life itself is a subtle thing and sustaining life is best achieved by travelling from the subtle to the obvious. Because life is really such a flimsy thing, its sustenance is best achieved by progressing from the simple to the great.

So when you are strong you can implement this and practise. But if you are weak, in order to sustain it you must first rebuild! For example, in spring nourish the spleen, in autumn nourish the liver, in summer nourish the lungs, and in winter nourish the heart.

You smelt the body so as to raise the fire, you return the Elixir to gather in the breath. This means using the passing months of the year – and not losing out on sustaining life.

> *NOTE: This is the One Rule in nourishment. We are reminded of more traditional methods of sustaining the heart and spirit, body, blood, breath and fluid-essences of the body. But they are not on their own a way of sustaining life. It is something quite separate from these activities. We need to travel from the subtle to the obvious, to follow the simple order of the natural world – in order to achieve greatness. Rebuilding is necessary if the energies are not strong enough to draw on for nourishment. This is spoken of later.*

It follows then that during spring and summer, we should sustain the Yang – using the True Breath to follow Heaven's Great Circulation, as it occurs within the liver and heart. It is the heart and liver that raise the breath upwards; and during autumn and winter we should sustain the Yin – using the True Breath to follow Heaven's Great Circulation, as it occurs within the lungs and kidneys. It is the kidneys and lungs that lower the fluid downwards.

spring and summer
sustain the Yang

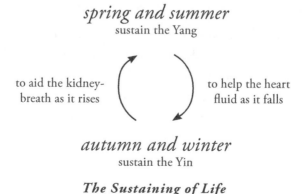

to aid the kidney-
breath as it rises

to help the heart
fluid as it falls

autumn and winter
sustain the Yin

The Sustaining of Life

This is to follow the turning about and transformation of Yin and Yang, the way not to miss out on the sustentation of life.

*NOTE: Sustain the Yang in the summer and sustain
the Yin in the winter. This is it, in essence. So then our
originating breath follows that of the sky: in summer it
is raised upwards and in winter it is lowered below. This
is to move along with the dalliance of water and fire.*

So when the kidney-breath is alive at midnight, and one Yang is born within the two Yin, at this moment 'quieten the mind and still the thoughts, close the eyes and straighten up the body, the fire of thinking returned to and starting up in the *dantian*'. This is its vapour being born and you with a method to sustain it!

And when the liver-breath is alive at dawn, and one Yang is born beneath the two Yin, at this moment 'sit alone and close the eyes, taking in more, letting out less, preserving the child and its mother in a deep embrace within the Yellow Room, creating a new-born little child'. This is the Yang being born and you with a method to sustain it!

So when the heart-breath is alive at midday, and a single Yin is born within two Yang, at this moment 'forget all speech and cease all thought, fill the mouth with saliva, held within, directly combating the heart-breath that it does not scatter, preserving the marriage of the Dragon and Tiger within the smoke and flame, so that then around the Metal Cauldron it playfully streams about and down below'. This is the *dantian* breath being born and you with a method to sustain it!

So when the lung-breath is alive at dusk, and a single Yin is born above the two Yang, at this moment 'close the eyes and dim the heart, concentrating on the region of the belly and side-ribs, preserving the Great Fire there burning within the cauldron, until there are Three Flavours within the cauldron, blazing upwards without cease, Three Flavours finally emerging'. This is the Yin being born and you with a method to sustain it!

So then eventually after three hundred days, the Foetus is complete and the True Breath of life finally born. Sustain this True Breath and smelt it 'to give birth to the spirit', the 'Five Breaths dawning at the First Gate', the 'Three Flowers gathering at the crown of the head'.

In five hundred days the Yang Spirit is born. Sustain this Yang Spirit and thenceforth smelt it, in order to join with those on the Path.

> *NOTE: The gist of the matter is just this – the kidney, liver, heart and lung-breaths. The 'fire of thinking returned', the 'child and mother in deep embrace', the 'dragon and tiger married amidst smoke and flame', the 'Three Flavours finally emerging', and the Holy Foetus and True Breath of life finally complete.*

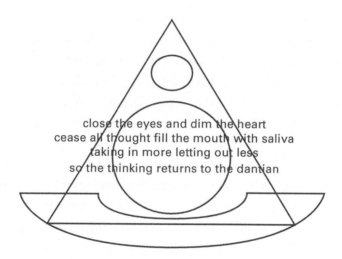

close the eyes and dim the heart
cease all thought fill the mouth with saliva
taking in more letting out less
so the thinking returns to the dantian

The Yang Spirit finally born

Once we are given a physical body, if we learn the art of sustaining it, we will give free rein to the True Breath of Heaven and earth in the human frame. It will arrive of its own accord – and once this living breath has arrived, if we learn to sustain it further, we give birth to the Model Dharma Body, the Astral Self; 'without the body, there is another body', and you transcend earthly matters to 'walk in the divine'. The Path of the sustaining life is, in brief, just this.

MIDDAY

the dantian breath being born

the heart-breath alive

the liver-breath alive   the lung-breath alive

DAWN   DUSK

the Yang being born   **the Yin being born**

the kidney-breath alive

the vapour being born

MIDNIGHT

NOTE: This chapter explains how after three hundred days the activity of sustaining the breath in all its aspects (Yin, Yang, dantian, etc.) is complete. The Foetal Breath may be also complete and the Breath of Life born. Sustain and smelt this living breath and it may be forged into spirit. 'Without the body, there is another body' and the Three Flowers of breath-energy, seed-essence and spirit then gather at the crown of the head. Eventually the Yang Spirit is born; smelt it and work further until finally you join with others on the Path. Then you, too, may 'walk in the divine'.

7

丹書

Sustaining the Body

…without the body there is another body, whereby we
may transcend earthly matters to 'walk in the divine'.

THE BREATH IS MOTHER TO THE MIND, THE BREATH
nestles in the body. Refine that breath and you capture the mind; it
follows then that refining the body enables you to find fulfilment in
the breath.

> If the Yang of the mind is not gathered in,
> Three Flowers cannot enter the Muddy Pill.
> If the True Breath has not yet fully dawned,
> Five Shadows cannot give birth in the Elixial Space.

This poem explains that without the body being 'caged up and
connected within', the mind and breath will lie apart.

> *NOTE: Notice the importance of the body. Sustain the
> body and it enables you to capture the breath. Refine
> this breath and you may capture the mind. The Three
> Flowers are the fluid-essences, breath and spirit. Essences
> refer to the body; breath to the breathing; spirit to the
> mind. The Muddy Pill is the brain. The Five Shadows
> are the Five Agents, fire, earth, water, metal and wood.*

The Yang of the mind makes up its clarity and strength. The Three Flowers consist of the fluid-essences, breath and spirit that constitute our human existence. The Five Shadows are the Five Messengers, fire, earth, water, metal and wood. These mix together the light and clear, the muddied and heavy.

Heaven and earth may be majestic, but they never escape the picture of the light and clear, the muddied and heavy; likewise, the sun and moon may be brilliant, but it is difficult to foretell their physical forms of roundness and brightness, the shaded and dark.

The accumulated Yang gives birth to the world as pure spirit, and the luminous sky rises above our heads, with its night-time stars and planets; the accumulated Yin gives birth to the world in physical form, and so beneath our feet appears the robust earth, with its stones and soil. Between them a steam or vapour rises up from the waters, forming into clouds and rain – this fluid then falling back down within the vapour, emerging as fogs and dew.

These myriad pictures crowd into life, and none lack a physical form – but it is only man who has an assembled spirituality that has donated him life, and it is he alone who must rely upon a Path in order to find fulfilment.

In this picture is the clue to sustaining your body. If you do not understand it, your fluid-essences and Po-soul will become scattered and wasted and the Yin Organs empty; before you are dead, your body will become like a dried-up piece of timber, and at the last gasp you are finished, ending up on the dung-hill of creation.

Now ponder deeply upon how to encounter the Path that enables you to sustain your body!

NOTE: What follows is simple homely wisdom.

THE *WESTERN MOUNTAIN RECORDS* STATE CLEARLY that during the second month of summer and the second month of winter, the best policy is to sustain the physical body, by dwelling in a deep hall, to avoid the breath of the great heat and great cold, and protect the muscles and flesh.

But this is not to be done too purposely. At the first cold put on warm clothing, but the clothing should not be increased too quickly; at the first warmth take it off, but neither should it be cast immediately away.

After a long period of work, rest and take your ease; this is to support the management of your strength; after a long period of inactivity, practise 'induction and conduction' (*daoyin* or stretching exercises), thus to circulate the breath through any stagnancies.

During warm summer days do not expose your body to the climate – exposure to the climate blocks up the life-force; in the summer do not sleep in damp places – sleeping in the damp scatters the breath and blood.

During cold winter days, avoid too much warmth. Extreme heat can mean the kidney Yang is weakened, and during the following spring and summer, the liver and heart may be attacked. During warm summer days, avoid seeking too much coolness. Extreme cooling can mean the heart is enclosed by a superficial cold, and during the following autumn and winter the lungs and kidneys may both incur deep blockages.

You should not wait for extreme hunger until you eat: eat but not to excess – excess food injures the spirit, whilst hunger harms the stomach. You should not wait for extreme thirst until you drink: drink but not too much – too much drink harms the breath, whilst thirst injures the blood.

Take a large wash every ten days, a small wash every five. Then our five breaths can stream around and circulate freely. A small wash means the life-force can move easily. In ten days our fate again returns. As the True Breath exists in the brain, if you wash the head properly, the eyes and ears will become sharp and clear.

If you take a small wash too frequently, the blood congeals and breath scatters, and although the body and flesh become bright and sleek, over a long period of time the breath is harmed. Then you suffer: for the breath cannot win over the blood, nor the mind win over the body.

Therefore the ancient peoples took the Yang in order to sustain the Yang, that the Yang did not wither and scatter; and took the Yin to refine the Yang, that the Yang did not weaken and become harmed. Then they followed this pattern year in, year out, day in, day out.

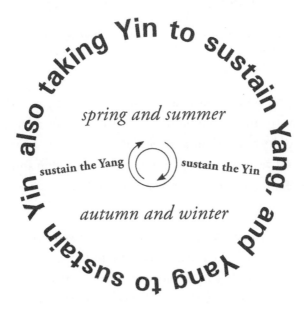

Spring and summer they sustained the Yang, autumn and winter they sustained the Yin, also taking the Yin to sustain the Yang and the Yang to disperse the Yin; during the single day, before midday they 'trained up the dragon' through the breath, so that at first it began to refine the physical body, whilst later it formed into the Gold Splendid; then after midday they 'trained up the mare' through taking medicines. If they did not have medicines, they were able to gather in the breath and refine an Elixir. If they could not do this, then they drew back the Fires of Desire in order to 'boil up the sea'.

MIDDAY

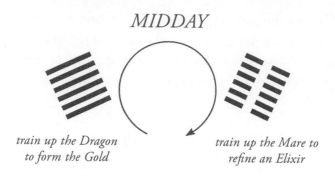

train up the Dragon   *train up the Mare to*
to form the Gold   *refine an Elixir*

All these approaches mean taking the True Yang as visible and working with it, inside the body – whilst if it is not apparent, then withdrawing the body in order to find it.

So then move into an empty room in order to sustain and complete the True Breath, letting it ascend within the body to extinguish the spooks of the Yin.

> NOTE: *Each day appears the same, yet all days are not the same. You must devote the utmost attention to 'responding to the moment'. Every season and time of the day you need to act accordingly.*

The Fellow who promotes this Path may have a broad view of many topics and have studied widely, but he only sustains weariness and failure if he mislays the general guide and pattern of Yin and Yang, and mistakes the path to the Silent Source.

The True Yin and True Yang together form the 'foetus', and they consolidate at the *dantian*; in a secondary sense, the True Yin manifests as the breath whilst the True Yang fashions our material body.

So now you have found it! 'Without the body there is another body', whereby we may transcend earthly matters and 'walk in the divine'.

8

Sustaining the Breath

...if you would retain your body, first sustain your
breath! Just as it is born sustain it, that it declines not.
Just as it weakens sustain it, that it disperses not.

HEAVEN AND EARTH MAKE USE OF CLARITY AND
turbidity in order to determine matter, and yet their energies must
be substantial enough to circulate around the Yin and the Yang; the
sun and moon make use of light and dark in order to separate out
physical form, and yet their energies must be sufficient enough to
join together our souls, the Hun and Po. This is stated in *The Secret
Book of Our Father*.

Together Yin and Yang, the Hun and Po, function as the pipes
and bag of a pair of bellows, being ruled by the out-going and in-
coming breath. These are the whole circumstances of the truth.

*NOTE: Here is neatly described the link between Yin
and Yang, the two souls of the Hun and Po, which
rest in the out-going and in-coming breath.*

'Wild birds may tumble about in the sky but they are governed by a
breath.' This is stated explicitly in *The Book of the Matching Shadow*.
They dive and turn in an empty space as if it were something solid.
Fish dart swiftly along but they are governed by the water through

which they swim. They move through the water as if it were empty space.

There are many trees that wither, and it is only the pine and cedar that stay hard and strong. This is because their sap-breath is able to remain firm within. Amongst the company of moving beasts that are destroyed by death, it is only the tortoise and crane that do not die. This is because their blood and breath are let be.

Their physical body becomes the refuge for a retained breath; this breath becomes the mark of a preserved body. Therefore if you would sustain your body and depart this world, first sustain your breath!

> Ultimately majestic and all-enduring,
> His breath blocks up all Heaven and earth!
> It gathers together as something divine,
> Roaming beyond the world of the senses.

Those most skilled at sustaining their lives learnt to sustain their physical bodies. Those most skilled at sustaining their bodies learnt by sustaining their originating breath.

THE *WESTERN MOUNTAIN RECORDS* STATE THAT throughout all ages those fellows who sustained their breath never escaped sickness, death or disaster, unless they were acquainted with the True Path.

In ancient times the population took a strong-minded fellow, who did not speak, to be one who could 'sustain his breath'. This indeed meant protection of the breath, but it was also to be lost in ignorance.

And people also take one who inhales the clean air and exhales the air that is stale to be one who 'sustains his breath'. This is to exchange the air within the lungs, but it is also to be lost in ignorance.

Those lost in dark ignorance, their breath scatters and their minds turn awry, their true spirit is daily suppressed and in the end it will never return. Those lost in dark ignorance, their *dantian* lacks any treasure. In vain they labour, spit out and suck in the common breath, but are unable ever to depart this world.

By 'breathing in more and breathing out less' you may be able to attack an illness – this is quite possible – but to describe it as the 'foetal breath' is a travesty of the truth. By 'swallowing above and returning beneath', you may be able to gather in a mouthful or two – again this is quite possible – but to label this as the Elixir of Return is a mistake.

Lao Zi has said: 'utterly gentle, as if hardly there at all; using it, without fail.' So they bow down before the breath and then they know the spirit. Every single breath, as it is about to leave they receive it in, not letting it out. Then they can close up the breath and refine the body. To 'gulp it down, and gulp it down again', to 'gather it in, again and again', both sides of the spine through 'deep breathing'. This is the so-called skill of 'forced irrigation'!

Or they 'sit up straight and raise the body, the breath filling the four limbs, the blood coursing through the veins, the whole body warm and comfortable'. This is the 'deploy the breath to incinerate the body'.

NOTE: None of these more crude methods is allowable.

All such methods as these are unsuitable. The Path of the sustaining of the True Breath is simply this.

> Just as it is born to sustain it,
> That it declines not.
> Just as it weakens to sustain it,
> That it disperses not.

For example, in the ancient employment of Hexagram 3 *Emerging*, which depicts a plant's shoot encountering resistance above, the Yang line, the 'nine at the first', is born, but still bent up and unextended; following this example, at dawn, you must embrace the image of an 'emerging shoot' in order to nourish your breath and make it strong. Also in the ancient employment of Hexagram 4 *Bubbling*, which depicts a spring of water bursting forth from under the mountain, the Yang line, the 'nine at the second' dwells amongst a flock of Yin lines, dark and unenlightened; following this instance, in the evening, you must embody its image and be just like a 'bubbling stream' in order to seek out the Yang and make it equitable.

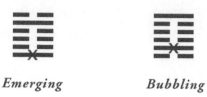

Emerging   *Bubbling*

NOTE: Strength is desirable in the morning; evenness in the evening. These examples are taken from my translation of the alchemical Cantong Qi, The Secret of Everlasting Life (Ch.1).

Now if you have a talent but do not energetically think it through, it creates trouble; if you have a strong will but do not attain energetic promotion, it makes for trouble; if you grieve excessively after suffering great distress, it creates trouble; if you rejoice and sing with too great a force, it creates trouble; if you frenetically give yourself over to desires, it creates trouble; if you weary yourself out with constant brooding, it creates trouble.

Perhaps you spend a long period laughing and talking, until sleep and rest lose out; or pulling the longbow or crossbow, or besotted with wine until you vomit it up, or filling yourself with food until you cannot move, or racing about until you are out of breath, or cheering out loudly or sobbing. Then Yin and Yang are disconnected, and accumulate great harm, so that soon you perish.

NOTE: In other words, moderation in all things.
'Just as it is born sustain it, that it declines not; just
as it weakens sustain it, that it disperses not.'

Those skilled at sustaining the breath remain in limpid calm, and eliminate all desire, dwelling in the quiet, solitary and alone, tending towards a view of themselves as 'rare and refined'.

In winter the Yang is born, and when the spring equinox is past, the Yang flourishes and the Yin disperses. At that time you should guard against any remnant Yin remaining in the belly and creating a sickness like bitter cold. In summer the Yin is born, and when the autumn equinox is past, the Yin flourishes and the Yang scatters. At that time you should guard against any remnant Yang remaining in the belly and creating a suffering like latent warmth.

> *NOTE: In other words, always be aware of the True Breath of Heaven and earth, the seasonal flux of warmth and cold, as it comes and goes. Seek to accord with the cycles of nature. Thus acupuncture treatment and herbal medicines are taken according to season.*

Do not look on the dead to protect against the deathly breath offending the living. Keep away from unclean places of refuse, lest the unclean breath offend the healthy.

When the True Breath is not yet robust and still bordering on weak, feed it constantly as it fills the mouth. When the True Breath is about to be severed but not yet gone, feed it constantly as it ebbs away.

In such a manner you may harmonise the breath, pacify the breath, disperse the breath, spit out the breath, gather in the breath, circulate around the breath, protect the breath and transform the breath: all these activities characterise methods by which you may sustain the breath.

> Your breath is like a silken thread,
> If you tug too hard, it is broken.
> It is like a wreath of smoke –
> Disturb it and it disappears.

Those who are unable to sustain the True Breath lose the method of protecting their body.

But to sustain the breath is not the same as 'capturing the medicine' and to 'capture the medicine' is not the same as 'refining the breath'.

As you capture the breath, you may 'return to source' and be able to form a Golden Elixir out of Yin and Yang; you may be able to refine it and 'exit the husk', moving on – in order to be transformed into a Winged Guest. However, before you can smelt this medicine, you must first capture it, and before you can capture it, you must first learn to sustain it!

9

心

Sustaining the Heart

That which takes responsibility for the world is the human heart…

MAN USES HIS PHYSICAL BODY AS HIS NEST WHILST HIS mind becomes its ruler. The mind must be close to the human heart. The book *On Penetrating the Mystery* states that when ruling the state, there is the division between prince and minister, whilst in the family, there exists the proper attitude of father and son. In our physical selves, the heart acts as prince or father, the breath as minister or son, whilst the body is as family or state.

> At the out-flowing of the heart's wishes,
> Nothing can stand in its way.

Amongst the Five Cycles in the natural world, the heart and mind relate to fire and to the southerly direction where the Yang is rich and abundant; amongst the planets it also corresponds to Mars.

> *NOTE: The heart stores up the blood which*
> *is red and warming. It is Yang, rich and*
> *abundant. Mars is the red planet.*

Its spirit is encountered like a 'red bird'. The body of the heart is shaped into three lobes or petals hanging downward, its colour like a bright red flower.

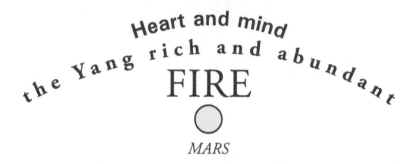

MARS

Its divine intelligence is quiet and obliging, transforming in an unfathomable manner, blending and merging together Yin and Yang. Its ideas are grand enough to encompass all that Heaven and earth produce, yet delicate enough even to enter into the smallest beard of wheat.

> Take control and they are correct,
> Let them go freely and they turn wild.

In this limpid calm, the Path is born; within any turmoil, the mind is lost. Simply remain empty and tranquil within and you will eternally support non-action. Then the body may turn resplendent.

Only when wildness 'jumps upon' resentment is it possible then to become a sage; only when a sage 'becomes lost' to resentment is it possible then to turn wild.

> *NOTE: The emphasis here is on the 'limpid calm' beloved*
> *of the Daoist sage or crafts-fellow. Take the story of*
> *Zhuangzi's butcher (see Zhuangzi Ch.3). The phrase*
> *'wildness jumps upon resentment' contains the character ke*
> 克 *meaning the control of desire. Between wildness and*
> *sageliness, resentment acts as a barrier to the heart.*

Throughout all ages the intelligent Fellow has sustained the reduction of his desires, in order to emphasise his true commitment. The True Source is then ultimately present; the magical brilliance lit up of itself, creating a lustrous shine – the Elixial Tower!

If you do not allow yourself to become bewildered by affairs, or damaged in a material sense, you may then well step out of earthly matters to 'walk in the divine'.

NOTE: This is our ultimate goal.

THE *WESTERN MOUNTAIN RECORDS* STATE THAT TO follow the Path and to be received into life is the task of our nature – whilst to embrace the One and be endowed with physical form is the task of our destiny.

That which takes responsibility for the world is the heart. That which recollects within the heart is the mind. That which creates thoughts in the mind is the emotion. That which stirs and expands the mind is the Hun-soul, whilst that which stills and contracts the mind is the Po-soul. That which flows into our bones and flesh makes up our blood. Those substances that strengthen our body and sustain our breath are the fluid-essences. A breath clear and alive is feeding us; a breath dull and heavy is being defensive. Being all-pervasive in every bone of the body it shows us what we are; appearing in many guises it gives us our physical shape. Acting stupid and obstructing others is just a matter of substance; being able to follow and go along with them is a matter of style. Separating out these two, the great and the small, is what gives us a human body.

NOTE: Our nature and our destiny need to be blended
– they need to work together as inner and outer in
all our affairs. This is our life: a question equally
of things biological, psychological and social.

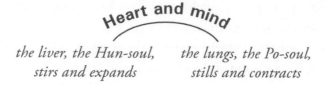

the liver, the Hun-soul,   the lungs, the Po-soul,
stirs and expands   stills and contracts

All our several thoughts unhindered are that which signifies the spirit; 'vast, boundless and ever-changing' signifies our spirituality.

The breath entering into the body signifies life; the breath departing from the body signifies death. Together these form a link leading our life onwards towards the Path.

The Path has a reality but lacks any form. It appears as nothing, yet contains the essence of life. Ever-changing, unfathomable, yet reaching the whole, it contains within itself both the spirit and flock of life.

The True People and Higher Immortals taught all people to foster the True Path that meant, at the same time, to foster the heart.

To teach people to foster the heart is to teach them to foster the Path.

The True Path cannot be seen, yet the heart illuminates it, so that, when and if the heart lacks constancy, it will be through the Path that it may be further retained.

> A humble heart banishes all fullness.
> A vacant heart is redolent with life.
> At its still-point without stirring,
> It becomes settled and immune from danger.
> The heart correct, it cannot be intruded on.
> When transparent, it may be without a stain,
> When pure it repels all uncleanliness.

These aspects of the heart are our birthright.

> The heart is straight and does not turn back,
> It is level within making distinctions.
> The heart is lit allowing no obscurity,
> It is made whole without a block.

These aspects of the heart are our birthright and in ordering them we will have enough in surplus.

> *NOTE: This passage forms the core of this important chapter. It states clearly that, in the province of the heart, humility is paramount. To foster the True Path is to cultivate the heart. Settled and still, it cannot be intruded upon. These aspects of the heart are inherent in our nature and, through according with them, we make our own reality.*

Seldom thinking, seldom considering, seldom craving, seldom working, seldom speaking, seldom laughing, seldom grieving, seldom delighting, seldom happy, seldom angry, seldom loving and seldom hating, we are able to keep the light of the heart from being shuttered.

In such a manner the spirit also remains uncluttered and this promotes the True Path of supporting life.

Alas! Those who misunderstand, they think too much and their minds are broken; they consider too much and their ideas are scattered. They crave too much and their breath is disputed; they are over-busied, which destroys their form.

Speaking out too much will weaken the breath, laughing too much harms the inner organs, grieving too much will consume the blood and delighting too much ebbs away the mind.

Too many pleasures break up the body, bit by bit. Too much resentment and the vessels of the body become untuned. Too much loving is close to being unprincipled. Too much hatred means you become haggard and lack a cheerful demean.

But the root-cause of all these troubles lies in allowing impurity into the heart, so that a harmonious breath is diminished by our own actions.

But if you are not able to sustain and lengthen your years, you will lose all cause for sustaining the heart.

The ancients said the heart and mind are like a pair of monkeys who are restless and can never keep still. They are just like two thieves who would rob you of all you have. Misfortune is certain!

10

Sustaining Longevity

Those skilled at longevity used the methods of fostering that 'which lies within'…

OUR FATHER AND MOTHER, THOSE TWO BREATHS OF Pure Yin and Pure Yang, take the seed-essences and blood to form the foetus in the Womb. Once the foetus is complete and the breaths sufficient, there forms a physical body. This is how a baby is born. This is duly noted in *The True Record of the Three Pure Ones*.

But this assemblage of magic relies upon there being a Path to follow. And then, as the mind and the breaths join together, the length of our lives is settled.

The very highest category of longevity lasts twelve thousand years. You protect the 'uncarved block' of simplicity and shoulder this utensil called life. Then, although you, yourself, may be lost and dispersed, the Path will never be lost.

The next best category of longevity lasts twelve hundred years. You retain a physical body but depart this dusty world. The Path remains, but the body remains also.

The lowest category of longevity lasts one hundred and twenty years. If you understand how to foster and refine your breath, you should be able to safely lengthen your years and attain this span.

But if you do not understand this method of refining your breath, your life will be gone, wasted and scattered; for you, yourself, are not the self you think you are. You are a 'circumscribed loner' that butts against the restrictions of life, which secretly and silently deduct from the count of your years. One count means three hundred days' extra life, one year of this and you nail your destiny! Twelve years and the record is complete. If you do not understand this and slacken in your work, it is because you take small evils as not hurting you. But they accumulate and will end in extinguishing your body. You may take small hurts as not harming you – but they will accumulate and eventually extinguish your life!

Then not even midway through your days you have already lost the greater part. The Higher Immortals and True People grieve and lament over this.

They have a method for escaping this world, but first you must have a plan for sustaining your longevity.

Investigate it and work at it and you are able to delay long enough to attain the highest longevity and sustain your life.

Do not shirk from this duty. You need to hold to it one thousand days. Then spontaneously you will find a track towards the Path that transcends this dusty world.

NOTE: An outline of the fabulous lives of the
ancients is given. We need to have time to foster
and refine our breath. Therefore we need longevity.
Without longevity, nothing is achieved.

THE *WESTERN MOUNTAIN RECORDS* STATE THAT YOU may understand the principles of sustaining life, but if you do not awaken to their practice, you will not live long. You may know and understand their methods, but if you do not know the ways of sustaining a long life, your cultivation will have no effect.

It is for this reason that those who would sustain their lives generally use prohibitions to protect their blessed lot.

Walk without saying much, lest the attention be lost and the breath harmed. Sleep without the mouth open, lest the breath escape and you diminish the spirit.

If you stand on the brink of a cliff, your Hun-soul leaps into your mouth. If you lie in a damp or draughty place, the breath will daily weaken.

You should not enter ruined temples or sinister shrines. Enter them and the peace of the mind is disturbed. Do not hunt for wild beasts. Attack them and the mind becomes frightened.

Spending too long outdoors under the Three Lights (sun, moon and planets) is to immerse your years and cut back on longevity. Bearing great weights on your back will almost certainly extinguish your destiny.

Drinking and feasting whilst next to sacred images, the Hun and Po-souls are not at peace. Sitting or sleeping close to graves or tombs, the mind is easily distracted.

You should not rest under great trees as this prevents the free movement of the human spirit. You should not float a boat in deep waters lest great cold obstructs the breath.

As flowers and grasses first emerge, do not cut them back, to prevent disorder from entering your home. If fruits are out of season, then do not eat them. This prevents evil sourness from entering the belly.

Never discourse with wild words or extreme opinions. Discussion diminishes man's power. Never mix fatty, sweet foods and wines. Mixing them harms the great body's root. Making light of slaughtering animals and things naturally does not yield a favourable birth.

High mountains should never be intruded upon. Entering them you will surely find misfortune. Beautiful objects should never be fondly coveted. Coveting them you will never find good fortune.

Harming people and things, wrong will repay wrong. Harbour enmity against the wise and capable, and resentment only breeds more resentment.

False teachings also discredit their teacher. These sorts of folk often have only themselves to blame – even though they learn clever rhymes by heart and meet with the curious and strange. The Great Path is then not undertaken – and beforehand you have wiped out your old age! You may use criminal ways and think you are about to get a good result – but actually there is no quick way to succeed.

> *NOTE: Simple folk wisdoms and maxims, in the Daoist manner. In the last paragraphs of this section, we begin to understand the purpose of this text. It is to refine the human spirit using simple means to become one on the Path, and to refine the Path in order to 'walk in the divine'. There is no 'quick fix'.*

Those skilled at longevity use the methods of 'fostering that which lies within' and through their principles are able to 'effect that which lies without'.

To 'foster that which lies within' is to secrete your fluid and seed-essences and to sustain your breath, to safeguard your Hun-soul and to cleanse your mind. Then the body and the mind may become altogether a mystery, and with Heaven and earth you may end your days.

You refine your spirit to be one on the Path and may step out of worldly matters 'to walk in the divine'.

To 'effect that which lies without' is to aid the needy and save the oppressed, to give help to all creatures and to benefit the people. Then there is filial piety within the family, loyalty within the state, obedience towards superiors and sympathy amongst the populace. Harm does not come to those who find gain, and nor do the over-worked seek out holiday times.

Generally follow the path of least resistance within your heart – never let others' opinions intrude upon you. Then you can begin to mobilise on the Path, more often than not coming across exceptional people.

Thenceforth you acquire the true method, until, once the work is in hand, you seldom meet with real problems and quickly acquire success!

However, although all the above may be achieved through self-cultivation, it may also be that the power of the Yin will try to consume you. If you cannot properly attain a sustentation of longevity, how will you ever then achieve wholeness?

The Rebuilding

11

Rebuilding Within

The Immortals and Sages of Old who cultivated this
truth always built within, they never built without...

IF YOU WOULD WISH FOR A LIFE UNENDING, TO DWELL
in Life Everlasting and depart this dusty world, then refine the fluid-
essences into a Magical Elixir and sustain their vital breath until they
turn spiritual. The True Immortals and Sages of Old who cultivated
this truth always built within, they never built without. *The Secret
Chart Depicting the Heavens* states:

> After the Three Pure Ones,
> Come the Three Great Ones.
> Within the Three Great Ones,
> Come the Two Manifestations.
> As the Two Manifestations separate,
> So appear the Five Ruling Powers.
> The Five Ruling Powers established,
> They unite in One Single Territory.

> *NOTE: The Three Pure Ones are Pure Clarity, Stillness
> and Quiet. The Two Manifestations are Yin and Yang.
> The Five Ruling Powers are fire, earth, water, metal and
> wood. The One Single Territory is the Single Domain*

> *of Life, built upon the fluid-essences – Heaven and*
> *earth, Yin and Yang, sun and moon, all together.*

Herein lie Heaven and earth. Above and below are displayed Yin and Yang, rising and falling, whilst from side to side the sun and moon come and go, shifting and turning.

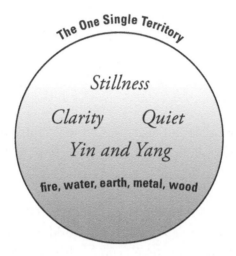

The One Single Territory

Stillness

Clarity   *Quiet*

Yin and Yang

fire, water, earth, metal, wood

They revolve about, returning and shifting their passage without it ever ending. They take on the image, the semblance of a ring, so that, to the end, there is no lapse in their progression.

And such is it within Man: with his fluid-essences as mother and his male breaths as lord. Amongst the Five Organs, each has its fluid-essence, and within each essence is born a breath. Amongst the Five Organs, each has its breath, and within each breath is born a spirit.

If you would wish for Life Everlasting, you need only learn to refine these essences into an Elixir, and sustain their vital breath until they turn spiritual.

> *NOTE: The Task is clear. Life is one continuous energy stream,*
> *with no break in transmission. It is the same in the common*
> *world as it is in each individual. Within the body, each organ*
> *contains a fluid-essence, a breath, a spirit. To dwell in Life*

Everlasting you need only learn to refine these essences into an
Elixir, and to sustain their breaths until they turn spiritual.

The Immortals and Sages of Old who cultivated this truth always rebuilt within, they never rebuilt without.

As what lies within becomes real and true, so that which lies without becomes workable.

Do not exert yourself at the impossible – work at that which comes easily and you will soon be rewarded. Then from out this common world you may 'walk in the divine'.

NOTE: See below how the human body is made. The Western
Mountain Records state this process quite clearly, outlining
the growth and development of the human embryo.

THE *WESTERN MOUNTAIN RECORDS* STATE THAT A MALE embryo first produces its right kidney, taking its essences without with its blood within, and the Yin being internally, whilst a female embryo first produces its left kidney, taking its blood without with its essences within, and the Yang kept internally.

NOTE: This is why a daughter is really also half-male,
carrying a Yang (male) within the Yin (female), whilst
a son is seen as also half-female, carrying a Yin (female)
within the Yang (male). This also explains the importance
of needing to extract the Yin from the Yang, the Dragon
from out the fire, and the Yang from the Yin, the Tiger from
out the waters, in order for them to be truly whole again.

The kidneys generate the spleen, the spleen generates the liver, the liver generates the heart, the heart generates the small intestine, the small intestine generates the large intestine, the large intestine generates the gallbladder, the gallbladder generates the bladder, the bladder generates the three source energies (fluid-essences, breaths and spirits), the three source energies generate the three burning-spaces, the three burning-spaces generate the eight vessels, the eight vessels generate the twelve major channels, the twelve major channels generate the twelve linking channels, the twelve linking channels generate the one hundred and eighty subsidiary collaterals, the one hundred and eighty subsidiary collaterals generate the one hundred and eighty other collaterals, the one hundred and eighty other collaterals generate the thirty-six thousand minute collaterals, the thirty-six thousand minute collaterals generate the three hundred and sixty-five bones, the three hundred and sixty-five bones generate the eighty-four thousand pores of the skin.

Once the foetus is complete, the breaths are sufficient, the spirit of consciousness enters into the body and it at once separates from its mother, becoming a separate individual.

In terms of inner and outer, the channels and subsidiary channels are internal and run within, whilst the muscles and flesh are external and exist without.

To sustain your life's destiny you must learn to sustain these inner organs. These great organs act as roots whilst, 'when the roots are strong, the leaves are healthy', of their own accord. To sustain your body you must sustain its five vital breaths, which lie within these organs. These breaths act as their source and 'when the source is deep, the current goes running outward', of its own accord.

> *NOTE: This is a description of the creation of the*
> *bodily form – as in 'the roots are strong, the leaves are*
> *healthy' and 'when the source is deep, the current goes*
> *running outward'. The yogic task is to rebuild the inner*
> *organs of the body, the treasuries of essences, spirits*
> *and breaths, the lungs, heart, kidney, spleen and liver.*
> *Then the roots are strong and the source is deep. How*
> *to carry out this task? The method is shown below.*

The Great Round of the True Breath follows the sky. The Small Round of the originating breath follows the day.

*NOTE: This depicts the macrocosm, with the True Breath,
during the seasons, rising and falling, and the microcosm, with
the originating or source breath of the day, coming and going.*

In spring the liver is prospering and the spleen is weak, so sustain your spleen by eating sweet foods, such as rice amongst the grains, the flesh of sweet fruits, the meat of oxen, etc.

Keep the mind clear and without fear. Fear injures the liver. Withdraw yourself and sit out the draught, because the liver detests a draught.

Every day make an interval at dawn to attend to the Small Round of the breath, and daily generate the source breath, sending it through into the liver.

> Stay vacant in mind,
> Remain unoccupied and cover the eyes,
> In order to sustain the liver breath.
> Over ten days you should see results,
> And your eyes become sharp and clear.

If you train in any lesser way, it will not have as good an effect.

In summer the heart is prospering and the lungs are weak, so sustain your lungs by eating spicy or pungent foods, such as yellow millet amongst the grains, the flesh of the cockerel, onions, etc.

Keep the mind clear and lessen your pleasures. Too many pleasures injure the heart. Sit quietly and out of the heat, because the heart detests the heat.

Every day make an interval at midday to attend to the Small Round of the breath, and daily generate the source breath, sending it through into the heart.

> Cut off all thoughts and rest at home,
> In order to sustain the heart.
> Over ten days you should see results,
> And the breath penetrate the hundred vessels.

If you train in any lesser way, again it will not have as good an effect.

In autumn the lungs are prospering and the liver is weak, so sustain your liver by eating sour foods, such as beans amongst the grains, plums and dog-meat, etc.

Quietly rest at home, to avoid the chill. If you get chilled, it injures the lungs. You should not express too much grief, because sadness injures the lungs.

Every day make an interval at dusk to attend to the Small Round of the breath, and daily generate the source breath, sending it through into the lungs.

> Position the body upright,
> Sitting quietly in order to sustain the lungs.
> Over ten days you should see results,
> And the muscles and flesh turn sleek and glisten.

If you train in any lesser way, again it will not have as good an effect.

In winter the kidneys are prospering and the heart is weak, so sustain your heart by eating bitter things, such as small grains, walnuts, lamb and mutton, etc.

Keep the mind clear and without any trepidation, because trepidation injures the heart.

Every day make an interval at midnight to attend to the Small Round of the breath, and you generate the source breath, sending it through into the kidneys.

> Withdraw the body and sit upright,
> In order to sustain the kidneys.
> Over ten days you should see results,
> And the *dantian* slacken of its own accord,
> The power of the breath energetic and strong.

If you train in any lesser way, it will not have as good an effect.

During the tail end of each season the spleen is prospering, so sustain your kidneys by eating salty things, such as wild rice amongst the grains, wild yam, fox meat and leeks, etc.

Settle the heart without any fear, because fear injures the spleen. Sit quietly away from the damp. Damp will harm the spleen.

Every day make an interval at early evening, early morning, just after midnight and just after midday to attend to the Small Round of the breath, and daily you generate the source breath.

NOTE: The practice is described in detail.

Now if the True Breath is allowed to become lost, the Fires of Desire will start upwards. Then the lungs open, the heart is in turmoil, the liver escapes out, the gall turns crosswise, all the ten thousand spirits are taken along with the true fire and blaze out. They abandon the body and roam around, the bones released, the tendons slackened and death advances on a single step.

> After a single loss, a single breath is weakened,
> After a hundred losses, a single spirit is gone,
> After a thousand losses, a single organ is gone.

Then in the end you reach the point of exhaustion, the four Great Limbs have no commander and you fall prostrate and dead.

Thus the True Immortals and Honoured Sages walked the Path of returning the essentially fluid forces of life, and as they set their whole mind upon the silent, originating source, they engaged the breath of the kidneys with that of the heart.

These accumulated breaths then generate a fluid, which, like a suspended pearl of dew, drop by drop, returns to the *dantian* (lower belly) and, if the 'timing of its firing' is not mistaken, condenses of its own accord.

> Its body like a crossbow pellet,
> Its colour the same as red lacquer.

Likewise 'within the breath is born a breath', and thus they refined the breath to fashion a spirit; again 'without the body is born a body', and they were able to transcend earthly matters so to 'walk in the divine'.

NOTE: This is the kernel of the alchemical process, as it starts to take place. Beginning as accumulated breaths in

the organs, these mixed breaths so generate a fluid. This
fluid condenses and returns back down to the lower belly.
The 'timing of the firing' means balancing Yin and Yang.

If you have not yet awoken to this clear humility, you are willingly turning your children and grandchildren into asses and oxen!

Perhaps the lascivious and depraved heart within you never ceases chattering – you should not involve yourself deeply in the Arts of the Bedroom. This is to avail yourself of shadows and appearances, to cheat the breath of the heart down into the Yellow Courtyard so that then the vapour of the kidneys is unable to rise up. Then you take 'the dragon revolving, the tiger turning over', desiring to forestall ejaculation and abandon your heart to false emotion.

In cases such as these, one tactic is to sit alone and withdraw the self, both hands enwrapped around the belly region. This causes the breaths to knot together. It is as if making your own foetus.

Another tactic is to sit the body up, the spine erect, withdrawing the attention a short while. This causes the breath 'at your elbow' to fly up into the brain! Repressing the blood into the brain, all the hundred bones will become filled, and you may defeat old age and experience again what it is to be young!

Also there are always those with only a slight interest in this task who lack awareness. They lust after capturing the juices and energy of some innocent girl or boy, in order to fashion a Shadowy Elixir; or else refine emotionless stones and minerals, taking the discarded breath of Heaven and earth to try fashion a material Elixir; or consume some herbal potions in order to rebuild the 'sea of the body's energies' within. If they are fortunate, they may partly succeed.

But all these mean you ultimately waste the breath and neglect your inner spirit. It means you turn your back upon the methods of the Spiritual Immortals and perpetuate a great lie. Those amongst you who are softly spoken will consider my words. Then who amongst you can go wrong?

12

补

Rebuilding the Breath

To rebuild the breath is the ultimate art…

ABOVE THE HIGHEST HEAVENS THERE IS NO DARKNESS, beyond the bowels of the earth there exists no light. From out the earth is born the Yang one hundred and eighty days and it ascends into the sky; but it does not pass beyond the sky. Thus the Yang light is born from within the Yin dark, as the silent breath of life, sending on down its surplus into the human spleen. These words come from *The Magical Texts Describing the Jaden Flower.*

> In a quiet room shut off the breath,
> 'Taking in more, letting out less',
> And 'in ten days you should see results',
> The body and limbs sleek and shining,
> The channels and collaterals lively and strong.

If you foster and develop any lesser art, it will never achieve a result such as this.

> *NOTE: The Yang life-force, the warmth of the spring,*
> *is born again from within the dark Yin world of the*
> *earth. The one hundred and eighty days comprise spring*
> *and summer. The surplus of breath is stored within the*
> *spleen. We need to follow this same art in the body.*

Each of the five inner organs has its season: one organ prospers whilst another weakens, one breath swells whilst another contracts. If you decrease where you find too much and build where there is insufficiency, once the organs are consonant together, all the joints of the body self-attune.

As all the joints of the body self-attune, all ails are stifled at birth.

Then as all ails are stifled at birth, a thousand harvests become a possibility!

> *NOTE: Again, following the ideas of the last few chapters, the admonition is to foster the breath – rebuilding where there is deficiency whilst reducing when there is excess.*

THE WESTERN MOUNTAIN SAGES STATE THAT THE breath ultimately has no form, and so must rely on having a semblance of existence within the physical body.

Once the physical body is formed, the breath is in place, and it can be fostered and built up: it matters not whether you are young or at the end of your life; what is valued most is the utmost devotion you give to this task, from beginning to end holding to the single aim.

> *NOTE: The task is the fostering and rebuilding of the breath, which exists within the physical body, notably the human spleen, in the manner described above. We must have the utmost devotion to this task, working steadily through the seasons of the year.*

The *Holy Rhyme on the Secret Usage of the Sacred Ruling Foetus* explained the highest doctrine of 'rebuilding the breath'. Bodhidarma's *Ultimate Principle of the Foetal Breath* also spoke of the middle doctrine. Later it was explained as 'foetal breathing' by Bian Que in the *Lingshu* and Ge Hong's commentary on *Foetal Breathing*. But these were of lesser importance. Beyond these there is nothing worth noting.

13

Rebuilding the Fluid-essences

> You must also understand the Path of rebuilding the
> fluid-essences: it is just the same as trying to guard a
> flame which is running out of oil.

THAT WHICH IS PURELY YANG ASCENDS AS THE BREATH,
whilst that which is purely Yin descends as fluid. This is quite clearly
stated in *The Hidden Mirror of Our Father.*

In such a fashion, the gaseous and fluid combine, and that which
pours into the space between the bones, collaterals and channels
forms into the bone marrow. As the gaseous and fluid combine, that
which emerges beyond the bladder forms the fluid-essences.

These essences reside severally within the five solid organs, the
heart, kidneys, liver, lungs and spleen; and the six hollow organs,
the large and small intestines, bladder, triple-warmer, gallbladder and
stomach.

Without the body these essences are reflected in the body hair,
flesh and skin, the hair on the head; eyes and ears, nose and tongue,
hands and feet; the blood and protective juices, the channels and
collaterals, and the various vital points occurring on the body and
four limbs.

As regards these essences, when the core of the breath resides in the liver, the liver itself produces an essence, and if this essence is not kept strong, the eyes dim and do not shine; as the core of the breath resides in the lungs, the lungs themselves produce an essence, and if this essence is not kept full, the body flesh becomes pale and weak; as the core of the breath resides in the kidneys, the kidneys themselves produce an essence, and if this essence is not kept topped up, the spirit of the body ebbs and lessens; and as the core of the breath resides in the spleen, the spleen itself produces an essence, and if this essence is not adequate, the teeth and hair on the head are less than strong.

> *NOTE: The heart and mind create a chamber for the core of the breath. The need is to keep the essences of the other organs strong. The best is daily practice.*

Amongst the five main organs, the kidneys act as a reservoir for the fluid-essences, just as the heart creates an open chamber for the breath.

The true seed-essences of the body reside in the kidneys, whilst any remaining essences themselves should return to the 'lower territory of the body'. The true energy of the body resides at the heart, whilst any remaining breath itself dawns at the central source, at the lower belly.

Thoughts, anxieties, worries and grievances all erode this breath. It is like gas escaping from the lid of a cooking pot. Wild or bad actions, disasters or disorder all take their toll upon the essences. They are like split twigs fed to fuel a blaze that is built up beneath the cauldron.

The Path of rebuilding these seminal essences does not solely consist in eliminating sexual desire – it also consists in being extremely cautious in all activity within the home. Be careful!

> *NOTE: We must persevere so as to preserve the breath and fluid-essences.*

THE *WESTERN MOUNTAIN RECORDS* STATE THAT HEAVEN and earth are stolen upon by the ten thousand creatures of this world, whilst all the ten thousand creatures are stolen upon by humankind. This idea comes from *The Book of the Matching Shadow.*

It follows then that the Yang ascends, the Yin descends – and all creatures receive the pure and unadulterated breath of the universe, the Yin forming their fluids and the Yang their flowering; and as mankind consumes these creatures, so he gives himself nourishment and fills himself within.

Everything we eat and drink is taken down into the stomach, mixing up with the True Breath and transmitted on and sent down into the Kidney Hall.

Now, this is how it happens. As a weakened breath begins to be amply filled, in the circumstances where it is born within the heart, if the heart-fire is *pressed down*, almost forced downwards, so that the vapour of the kidneys cannot ascend, then 'to the left it turns, to the right it revolves', and the intercourse of the Dragon and Tiger begins.

This is just how it happens in the natural world whilst when the mature Yang is supporting the foetal Yin (at midsummer) the Yang is also doting upon the fading Yang, and the Yin is forced up against the Yang. Now from the sky the Yin is coming down, and in one hundred and eighty days it reaches the earth.

Likewise, as the Yin passes over the earth, the Yin carries within itself the vital Yang (at midwinter), the Yin wrapping itself around the substance of the Yang. But the Yin is also doting on the fading Yin and the Yang is forced up against the Yin. So then from within the earth the Yang begins again, circulating around and returning back, and they join up together without missing step.

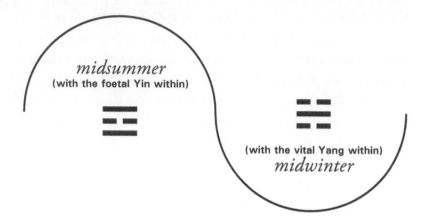

NOTE: The Book of the Matching Shadow states 'heaven and earth plunder all things, all things plunder man, and man plunders all things.' Heaven and earth steal upon the passage of Yin and Yang in order to form the breath of the seasons. This is an example of rebuilding.

In addition, within the body there is the transference of the 'stirring thunder' as when one lies on one's side calmly, in meditation. The loins of the human body correspond to an area of water, and when this water is still, there is born a fire; it emerges like a rising mist, like a silken thread. If you disturb it, it is broken; if you rub it out, it is gone.

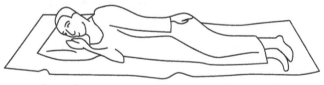

when the water is still, there is born a fire

The eyes, ears, nose, tongue, body and mind are the six wants that injure us without; happiness, anger, grief, laughter, love and hate, and moping are the seven states that injure us within.

Up above the Many-Storied Pagoda has fallen and gone – down below the Golden Turtle has been cast away and lost! Then it is like throwing out a broken net to catch the wind – you will never succeed!

Certainly you must understand this Path of rebuilding the fluid-essences: it is just the same as trying to guard a flame that is running out of oil. Now count the days until you will return to enter the Circle of Transmigration!

14

Rebuilding a Surplus

Even though you are of tender years, you can still arrive at depletion.

THE PATH OF SUSTAINING OUR LIVES TAKES 'AVOIDING depletion' as its main aim, whilst the Art of prolonging our lives makes 'rebuilding' a priority. Dwelling at peace and thinking on any future catastrophe, you may guard against the unseen. This is stated in *The True Book on the Cave of the Spirit.*

Therefore do not consider small dislikes as unharmful, but avoid them – and do not consider small joys as unhelpful, but welcome them.

Rise in the morning and retire in the evening. Let your rising and retiring be early or late, according to the four seasons; let your activity and rest always be controlled by the rule of creating an overall harmony.

To attune the tendons and vessels, there is no better method than 'bending and stretching' the body; to sustain the healthy energies and cast out the old, there are the physical arts of 'spitting out and taking in' the breath; to circulate about the life-blood and energy, there are the skills of 'building up and knocking down' where there is insufficient or excess; to regulate your daytime work, there is the code of give and take.

Take a restraining hold on your anger and it will round out the Yin breath, whilst setting a curb on pleasures will sustain the Yang breath. Use clear humility to escape errant thoughts, whilst you practise quiet contentment to sustain the soul.

> *NOTE: It could not be said better. Daoism*
> *is a religion of keeping quiet.*

Even though you are of tender years, you can still arrive at depletion: the breath weak and the body wretched. An older person should now understand this, and investigate how to protect against any suffering to build up a surplus of energy within.

> Take the breath to rebuild the breath,
> And the breath itself suffices;
> Take the spirit to refurbish the spirit,
> And the spirit will be in abundance.

As the breath fills out, so the body lives longer. As our spirit flees this dusty world, so our life and destiny are naturally prolonged.

THE *WESTERN MOUNTAIN RECORDS* CLEARLY STATE THAT: Whosoever follows the True Path, Heaven will not destroy! Who swallows the Silent Breath, the earth will not extinguish.

This suggests taking the ultimate Path as one's neighbour, whilst understanding that it can also coexist within one's own body.

Keep the heart pure and simple, and your destiny is prolonged naturally, without end.

The Indictment on the Six Secrets says that anyone who desires to acquire Life Everlasting should foster that which engenders life, beginning with the fluid-essences and breath.

Both the fluid-essences and breath coalesce to fashion a human body. This body is fundamental to receiving life, whilst the breath makes up the foundation of the body.

A popular saying is 'In the morning train up the dragon, after midday train up the mare'.

A Yang breath is born from within the kidneys: at the midnight hour is its beginning, at the midday hour its end, and so it ascends and prospers.

For this reason 'train up the dragon of Qian', meaning to sit up quietly in an empty room, close the eyes and dim the heart, raising up the body without stirring, causing the breath to fill out the four limbs, to steam up and waft throughout the body, the life-blood and energy moving freely.

After many days this breath may be abandoned and the spirit will become clear.

As well as this, when the vapour from the kidneys reaches the heart, the accumulated breaths generate within themselves a precious fluid. A Yin fluid is borne from within the heart: at the midday hour is its beginning, at the midnight hour is its end, and it descends and prospers.

For this reason 'train up the mare of Kun', meaning to close the eyes and dim the heart, withdrawing the body whilst sitting upright, taking both hands to enclose the belly, sinking the heart-fire down into the *dantian*, to boil up the sea of breath within.

After many days this breath prospers and the spirit will become clear. This is to build up a surplus of breath.

> *NOTE: Yang vapour is born out of the kidneys; Qian is the trigram of the Yang-heavens; Yin fluid is born from the heart; Kun is the trigram of the Yin-earth.*

in the heart is born a Yin fluid

*train up the
Dragon of Qian*   *train up the
Mare of Kun*

in the kidneys is born a Yang vapour

In winter avoid the cold, in summer avoid the heat; in cold weather avoid the wind, on hot days avoid the sun.

In labouring do not weary out the body or limbs. When at rest do not idle away the flesh and muscles. Every five days take a small wash, every ten days a large wash.

When the breath is weakening, do not be active. When the blood is prospering, do not rest. This is to build up a surplus of breath.

Perpetually sever all lusts and desires in order that they do not stir up the heart. This is the best course. In their stead, foster the truth in other ways and words. Because of the occurrence of death, seek life!

Although the physical body engages in sexual intercourse, the breath must not engage in intercourse; although the whole person may be coarse, still the physical body should not be coarse. Do not think just of yourself, relate to your wife also – but never allow any undue loss.

When you suddenly feel the need for undue emotion, pull back and out, cheating the mind of its power – to rebuild the Silent Source below. Then you can settle your inner nature and life. This is the next best course.

At thirty years old, Yin and Yang attract each other, and you can never escape the feeling for sex. It is suitable every five days, one measure; at forty every ten days, one measure; at fifty each twenty days, one measure; at sixty once a month, one measure; at sixty-four you may divine the end of your years. So then there is no need to speak any further of measures.

> *NOTE: This is quite simply a formula for limiting the loss of sperm in the male. Women can draw their own conclusions. Sexual excess seems less likely in the female.*

If you ennoble and pay homage to the Silent Source, and desire to seek Life Everlasting beyond death, you should not criticise this view. It enables one to build up a surplus of fluid-essences.

To build up the physical body is not as good as building up a surplus of essences; to build up a surplus of essences is not as good as building up a surplus of breath; to build up a surplus of breath is not as good as building up a surplus of spirit.

If you build up the spirit, both the body and breath will be eternally secure.

From time immemorial, for the intelligent fellow there has never been much discussion about the possession of a surplus on the spiritual Path. Frequently one sees no effects outwardly whatsoever. It demands nothing special beyond the total devotion and commitment of the inner spirit to its main cause!

In ancient times True Man Liu Gang, on a certain day and at a certain time, was blessed with both a healthy body and sound spirit. He gained the spirits of all gathered together and found Life Everlasting beyond death. Likewise the exceptional fellow Bian Que sat still in his own house, in an empty room, harmonised his spirits and 'exited his husk'. Like a strong man flexing his forearms, he could walk a thousand, even ten thousand, miles.

> NOTE: *Here for the first time we hear of an adept who could 'exit his husk'. He is the legendary doctor Bian Que, renowned as one of the earliest exponents of acupuncture. He is said to have written the Lingshu, or 'needling classic'. By 'exiting his husk' he could acquire another body. 'Without the body, there is another body.' This is the so-called 'astral body'.*

If the Yin-soul dare not oppose you, you may still retain your body and depart this dusty world. Moreover you may build up a scattered magical breath all for yourself, and also benefit, with respect, the Hun-soul and spirit.

Human happiness and catastrophe can possibly be foreknown. It comes down to the magic of the spirits. When death and life are both eternally cast out, there remains only the One Truth and reality.

As we progress further along this path of rekindling the spirit, we approach closer to both the clarity of the self and the sustaining of life. This implies the ceasing of thought and the quieting of the mind. Thereafter both movement and rest are in perfect accord, one's progress responds in measure, the Elixir is finished, and the breath of life, of its own accord, turns out true.

Once your breath runs true, you naturally have all the spirit you need. A genuine surplus indeed!

15

Rebuilding Depletion

A life without undue inebriation; an evening without going astray; this is the best scheme for rebuilding depletion.

THE YIN DARK WITHOUT A GLIMPSE OF LIGHT MAKES for a disembodied being; the Yang light without a shade of dark makes for an immortal; light and dark mixed heterogeneously make for a human soul. This fact is quoted often in *The Scattered Records of the Ten Realms*.

A disembodied being follows the dark Yin magic of the breath; as this breath condenses, so a being is given shape. An immortal fellow follows the bright Yang mellifluence of the breath; develop this breath, without it scattering, and it will attain substance.

In the human soul, when the Yang bright is exhausted, the self becomes a disembodied being – a disembodied being is that to which we may all once return. But as the Yin dark is exhausted, the self finds immortality – an immortal being is that into which we all may once be transformed.

> *NOTE: Note the clear distinction between Yin and Yang, the disembodied and the immortal, the dark and light. The life-force is the Yang. The death force, the Yin.*

Those of tender years, when the Yang is plentiful and the Yin still unformed, if they are not willing to develop and train up their Yang, they will become old and feeble.

After your breath is scattered and gone, how can you best rebuild this depletion? The high-minded fellow and best students work steadily, even when they have not as yet rebuilt anything, and guard cautiously what they have built, even once they have sustained depletion.

Before depletion is present, you must support and sustain your vigour – that you may turn depletion aside; once depletion is present, you should rebuild a surplus of vigour – that you may not sustain harm.

But if you shun the high-minded and neglect to tread the Noble Path, you will not be up to this.

THE *WESTERN MOUNTAIN RECORDS* STATE: OUR HUMAN form receives its vital breath and steals itself a body; within three hundred days the foetus is fully formed and separates from its mother; one thousand days, it suckles at the breast; four thousand days, it plunders the material substance of this world, fulfilling the plan of its destiny; until at five thousand days it is fully formed and complete.

Therefore, when a girl approaches her fourteenth year, her natural menses descend and her True Yin force is broken and scattered. When a boy approaches his sixteenth year, his true seed begins to fill and the Yang energy on its first occasion leaks out. This is to incur natural depletion. How many more times does this have to happen – if you do not understand the nature of fostering the development of Yin and Yang and their natural sustentation!

For example, in the halls of the Kings of Old, there were beautiful women, troops of handsome lads, male servants and female handmaidens by the thousands. By day they leaked out their marrow, in drunken revels; during the night they transported the blood into their veins, closeted in the bedchamber, their eyes and ears filled with sensation; in bed, supposedly asleep, but never securing rest; dillying, dallying but never at peace, taking stimulating foods, lying on silken covers, and entering the bedchamber highly inebriated.

Never did they understand the harnessing of the spirit or the breath. They lived a life without restraint and their seed-essences and minds were crippled and obstructed. Then not even halfway on to one hundred years they were already burnt up, withered and lost.

The Ancient Sages and True Immortals generally made use of this practice of sustaining the Yang. Even if they had a surplus of energy, they still only sought to be without depletion. A life without undue inebriation, an evening without going astray, or a night without excessive activity in the bedchamber. This is the best scheme for rebuilding depletion.

In a similar fashion, man cannot exist without the five tastes, but one should guard against having too great a preference. Sour tastes deplete the spleen, sweet tastes deplete the kidneys, salty tastes deplete the heart, bitter tastes deplete the lungs and spiciness depletes the liver.

There are no such great medicines as your own hunger and thirst – although you should eat three meals a day. The ancient peoples made a point of eating bland foods. Also they did not eat strong-tasting stuffs or meats, lest they defile the mouth and belly.

If the five organs have built up obstruction, then you may use the Method of the Six Character Breaths to heal them. This is a method derived from the *Map of the Yellow Courtyard*. By these means you can heal any disease and lengthen your days. Furthermore, you may then be able to foster your own physical self – in order then to heal others.

The secret of the Method of the Six Character Breaths is simple. It lies in following the seasons: 'in Spring not to over-exclaim (*hu*), in summer not to over-smile (*shen*), in winter not to over expel the breath (*he*), in autumn not to over-sigh (*xu*).'

If each and every one of these breaths is respected in season, and throughout you constantly retain these 'small cries', then the 'three burning-spaces' (torso) will never encounter insufficiency. If during all the eight festive periods you not over-puff yourself up, then the Kidney Hall will have no trouble in filling.

This is also to follow the popular saying:

> In excess, guide the child;
> In deficiency, kill the devil.

This additional secret nobody ever understood. It was only the Ancient Sages of Western Mountain who acquired some experience in this matter.

It is not necessary to have one hundred rules or prohibitions: only 'at dawn not to be empty, in the evening not to be full', this is the best rule. In other words, eat more at the beginning of the day.

'To eat plainly without strong tastes and blandly without strong meats' is the next best rule. Why then worry about the body and limbs not having enough or being happy?

NOTE: What follows now is the use of the Birth and Control cycles amongst the Five Elements to rebuild depletion.

In the Method of the Six Character Breaths, the saying 'in excess, guide the child' and 'in depletion, kill the devil' works thus: the liver's original sound is *xu*, so, if there is excess in the liver, use *xu*; if *xu* is still unable to guide the liver-breath, perhaps then 'guide the child', that is, use the *he* character to drain the excess breath of the heart; once the breath of the heart is moving, the breath of the liver will turn around of its own accord ('fire is fed by wood').

If the liver itself is depleted, then 'kill the devil': this refers to the lungs. The gold of the lungs is conquering the wood of the liver, making the wood the wife and the gold the husband: the husband then is the 'devil'. If the breath of the liver is weak, it must mean also that the lungs are in excess, so in this case it is necessary to 'kill the devil', using the *shen* character (from the heart) to eradicate the disorder in the lungs ('fire conquers gold').

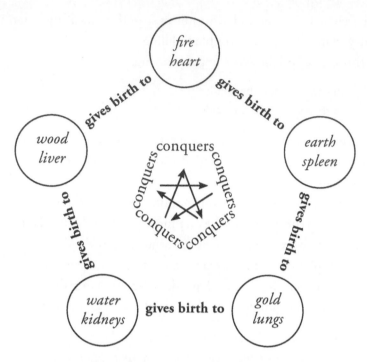

The Governance of the Elements

The fellow of supreme wisdom examines his own intelligence in order to understand the 'birth and control cycles of the Five Elements'. He blends together their differing breaths, providing neither too little nor too much, so that Yin and Yang, of their own accord, are corrected and agree.

As you match with the seasons and festive periods, you simply 'drop your hand' and the whole work progresses; you gain a tacit understanding of the Workings of Heaven through being totally immersed in their silent rule.

How then can Life Everlasting not be achieved? How then will a Fairy Immortal not be made!

> *NOTE: The other great truth is that we can use one taste to combat another, one foodstuff to ameliorate the effects of an invading taste; for example, if you eat too much*

*sweet, do not try to combat it by reducing sweetness;
rather eat more sour, salty, etc. The function of herbal
medicines is primarily to correct taste imbalances.*

The Verification

16

水火

The True Water and Fire

...taking Yang as its role, whilst hiding in its midst
a single sliver of the True Yin; taking Yin as its role,
whilst hiding in its midst a single sliver of the True
Yang.

THE YIN GENERATES WATER AND WATER IS NATURALLY
cooling, but there is a warm Fountain of Golden Sunlight immersed
within the water, so it is never fully cool. The Yang generates fire and
fire is naturally heating, but there is a chill flame on the Mound of
the Mournful Marsh facing the fire, so that it never funds more than
a gentle warmth. This is the text that comes from *The Secret Rhyme on
the Yellow and Central*.

> *NOTE: In the external world, water as rain, pond,
> sea or marsh is always lit by the fire of sunlight, so it is
> never completely cold. This is the 'warm Fountain of
> Golden Light'. Flame and fluid interact; fire and water
> act together in life, always. The chill flame probably
> refers to marsh lights, naturally occurring methane.
> This is the 'chill flame on the mournful mound'. These
> examples exactly describe this process in nature.*

Thus, if water and fire lying without the body have it in their minds to invert and interact, as Yin and Yang also lie within the physical body, how can you keep them from turning to each other!

For instance, the kidneys represent water, but within the waters is born an energy, this energy actually consisting of fire; the heart represents fire, but within this fire is born a fluid, this fluid actually representing water. This is the fire within the water and the water within the fire.

The fluid is able to irrigate all the body's vessels, whilst the fire can waft through the four limbs. Water and fire in humankind act in just such a fashion.

> *NOTE: Thus continues the discussion of internal*
> *alchemy, the intricacies of Yin and Yang, water*
> *and fire, water in fire and fire in water.*

AS SOON AS THE ULTIMATE SOURCE IS DIVIDED IT creates the two powers of Heaven and earth. This is the point discussed in *The Discourse on the Penetrating Silence.*

> Heaven takes the path of Qian.
> Light and clear, and positioned above,
> It takes the Yang as its role;
> Hiding within its midst
> A single sliver of the True Yin.

This is because, after the winter solstice, the Yang warmth ascends from in the earth, until by the summer solstice it has arrived at the heavens – the accumulating Yang of which then gives birth to the Yin. The Yin generally attracts more and more Yin to it, without being lost: dispersed, it forms into mists and condensed it forms the dew, until a vapour of mist and dew emerges out of the heavens. This is the Yin and true water.

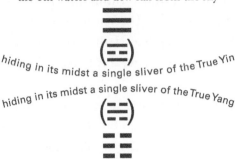

after the summer solstice,
the Yin waters and dew fall from the sky

hiding in its midst a single sliver of the True Yin

hiding in its midst a single sliver of the True Yang

after the winter solstice,
the Yang clouds and rain emerge from the earth

The True Yin and Yang, Born in the Outside World

Earth takes the path of Kun.
Heavy and turbid, it is positioned beneath,
Positioned beneath, it takes the Yin as its role;
Hiding within its midst
One single sliver of the True Yang.

This is because, after the summer solstice, darkness falls from the sky, until by the winter solstice it arrives on the earth. This is the accumulating Yin that gives birth to the Yang, the Yang generally attracting more and more Yang, without being lost; as it ascends it forms clouds, and as it disperses it forms rain. In such a fashion the energy of the clouds and rain emerges out of the earth – as the Yang and true fire.

> *NOTE: This is the Yin appearing within the Yang*
> *and the Yang appearing within the Yin, during the*
> *passing of the seasons. Qian and Kun are the male*
> *and female, purely Yang and Yin, trigrams.*

Within the human race it is all just same; at the very beginning, in the very foetus, we receive the seed-essences from our father and the blood from our mother: these two energies join together.

The Yang-type energies rise above, the heart establishing itself as the 'palace of the breath', whilst within this breath is concealed a true fluid positioned at the heart. The Yin-type energies fall beneath, the kidneys establishing themselves as the 'abode of the waters', whilst within these waters is concealed a true breath, positioned between the kidneys.

If we had not been created in such a fashion, how could the breath of the kidneys ever reach out to the heart? And how could their accumulated energies ever give birth to a fluid – a single Yin born within a double Yang? On the other hand, how could the breath of the heart ever reach down to the kidneys, and their accumulated fluids give birth to a breath – a single Yang born within a double Yin?

> *NOTE: Microcosm, macrocosm; it is all the same. In the outside world, Yin is born within Yang at midsummer, and Yang within Yin during midwinter. Similarly there is a midsummer and midwinter within; we are just a small universe. In this small universe water and fire admix, just as do the seasons outside. Water flows down and fire blazes up. The cooling Yin mists and dews come into the empty skies in autumn time. This is like the true watery fluid born out the Heart-fire, the Yin fluid born in the Yang as in the trigram Li-fire. Similarly the fertilising Yang produces clouds and rain out of the earth in spring time. This is just like the true fire coming out of the water, the Yang vapour born from between the Yin kidneys as in the trigram Kan-water. In the human form, water is needed to cool us above, whilst fire must be sent down to warm us beneath. The true fire below and the true water above are a symbol of 'all being complete'.*

Hexagram 63 – All Complete

THERE ARE DIFFERENT TYPES OF FIRE AND WATER. THE *Western Mountain Records* clearly indicate that water's existence is just because one breath spreads and sends out to another breath – and these accumulated breaths then generate a fluid. So this means each of the five organs has its own fluid. This is called the 'fleshy water'.

But as well as the 'fleshy water', there is the 'true water', the 'spiritual water' and the 'Dharma water'.

When the water of the True One lies concealed within the kidneys it is the Yin Tiger, or 'true water'. Again the instant the fleeting Gold Material enters the Upper Palace and turns below from above, running up against the true fire and producing the conditions of *Once Succeeded*,[1] with fire below and water above, this is called the 'spiritual water'.

Then again, when perhaps you are sick, and you close the mouth to draw in a mouthful of breath at a time, one mouthful at a time – then if you convey the breath to where the disease occurs, any problem will heal. This is called the 'Dharma water'. Water has such many and varied uses, their characters are all different.

The moment the True Breath is born, it is due to be watered and irrigated, using the rule of 'washing and bathing'. You smelt the body so that the True Breath rises, then returns and comes back. This is because of the rule of the Elixir of Return.

Master 'Sea Toad' said:

> Twin Glories, they mark out
> The Jewelled steps to the Temple,
> A Great Ditch releasing
> Eight bowls of Nectar Wine.

This is a clear indication of the Jaden Fluid Elixir of Return.

Duke Lu has said:

> As Water and Fire arrive
> At their moment of Union,
> The trigrams' completion
> Tidies up both Heaven and earth.

---

1   Hexagram 63, also known as *All Complete, Already Over.*

> One rises and the other falls,
> The Yang smelting the Yin.
> The moment the Yin is gone,
> Such significance! A hidden truth!

This is to describe the work of water and fire, one above, one below, again, the timing of *Once Succeeded* (Hexagram 63).

And the 'Freely Wandering' Master said:

> The Dharma water can arrive at the Hidden Gate!
> It freely wanders through, all day and night
> Sent all around in a ring...

This is explaining how the 'Dharma Water' can be a true agent in healing disease. For the most part, the above explain the most common uses of water.

> *NOTE: 'Tidying up' is a reference to All Peaceful*
> *(Hexagram 11), where the Pure Yang is below and*
> *the Pure Yin above. Water and fire, water above, fire*
> *below, are timed into their correct positions in Once*
> *Succeeded (Hexagram 63). 'Sent all around in a ring'*
> *signifies the breath surrounding totally the body.*

There are also different types of fire. The bladder forms the 'people's fire', the kidneys form the 'ministerial fire', the heart forms the 'monarch fire'. Yet there is also the 'fire of ignorance', the 'Elixial fire' and the 'total body fire'.

In general when you do not understand something or somebody, and are harassed by things, angry or frightened, this represents the 'fire of ignorance'. This is the first type of fire.

Again, when you learn to lower this fire and send it down to heat up the *dantian*, the mind held as one and unshaken, guarded with the utmost ease and devotion, this is using the fire to heat up and smelt the Elixial Medicine. This is called the 'Elixial fire'.

Again, when the fire rises up and then returns back downwards at the rear of the body to start passing through the Double Gates, this illustrates the Chain-and-Bucket Water Pump. Then the fire rises up the front of the body, and crosses out through the Many-Tiered Building (torso), where it forges and smelts the material Yin; once it has passed both front and back, filling out totally the body and limbs, it incinerates the whole self. This is the last type of fire, the 'total body fire'. For the most part, the above explains the most common uses of fire.

> *NOTE: The Double Gates are the kidneys. The*
> *Chain-and-Bucket Water Pump, or River Pump,*
> *has been described previously in Chapter 5.*

There is a secret stated by the Sages of the Western Mountain in *The Book of the Nine Immortals.* It says:

> In small troubles, use water.
> With great troubles, use fire.

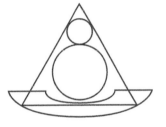

If perhaps a trouble is great, its root lies in inconstancy. Perhaps the self is troubled and cannot find peace. Immediately enter a quite room, let down your hair and loosen your clothing; close the eyes and dim the heart, sit upright and hold the position firmly. This is because 'a raised body promotes the fire'. So then you must *slightly retain* the breath.

> Briefly taking it in,
> Slowly letting it out.

As you silence the thoughts and place them beneath the navel, a fire revolves in the space of a tenth of a bushel and instantly a flame rises within the body. It can perhaps be compared to a turning screen or flowered canopy, shading and settling your whole body, protecting you and ensuring that Yin devils and evil sprites dare not approach.

> *NOTE: A tenth of a bushel is about 1 dm². The flowered*
> *screen or canopy can be seen to occupy the space around*

> *the heart and lungs of the body. This screen protects them*
> *from evils. In ancient times a decorated canopy protected*
> *the Emperor whilst he made his tour of the regions.*

Buddhism speaks of quelling the fire Mara, the lord of demons; Daoism describes a fire burning up within the body. Both employ the image of a flaming fire to stress shutting off both passions and sexual desires, over a long period of time – that the source of the Elixir may be solidly determined. If this seems at all impossible, then introduce water and fire to each other, and the Dragon and Tiger will go at it – in order to complete an Elixir!

Once the Elixir is finished, the Yin Spirit Realms will scatter of their own accord and dare not approach, whilst the Yang Realms, quite naturally, are unwilling to depart.

Once the Yang spirit is present, the physical body becomes stronger, the Yin retreats and the breath-energy is retained as one. Once the energy is retained as one, the body will become whole and firm, and you are naturally able to mature into living a fuller life.

17

龙虎

The True Dragon and Tiger

...the water of the True One, the Yin Tiger; the vapour of the Proper Yang, the Yang Dragon...

THE TRUE DRAGON AND TIGER, WHERE THEY LIE AND may be engaged, has been kept a secret and never disclosed, at any time. It is only in *The True Book of Great Unity* that the state of their supreme marriage is revealed. This is how it is stated in *The Alchemical Book on the Dragon and Tiger*.

In two books, *The Source Revelation of the True One* and *Strange Words Spoken by One Encountering Enlightenment*, there is also a clear reference to the mystery of the Dragon and Tiger.

One view is that they lie in the Five Wildernesses of the Kun-lun Mountains; another within the Great Gulf of the Northern Pole, 'concealed in a jaden case, engraven with golden letters, sealed with a golden wax, stamped with a jade insignia, attended by fierce officials, and holy men standing by'.

Deny all affinity with this dusty world! And at last you might begin to understand these few words.

The True Fellow 'Great Purity' says –
Craft the Five Powers topsy-turvy
And a Dragon comes out the Fire;
If the Five Powers are not let free
The Tiger is born out of the Water.

A slight rule indeed! But a magic rule: simply, pure magic! Thus the catch to the silent workings of the Universe may be undone.

Duke Lu has it from his book written on *Peering into the Mirror of the Medicine* where we hear about the ground of the human heart 'turning clear'. The Yang Dragon is said to emerge from out the fire, whilst the Yin Tiger is born again out the water.

Both creatures on this occasion provide a basis for the Path. Once each region has been traversed, you finally gain the title 'Elixir'. If you foster this truth supremely and understand it all, you will easily mount the Red Dragon to revisit the Jade Capital!

Again, the book *Peering into the Mirror of the Medicine* reveals that 'a breath is born from within the kidneys' and that within this breath is hidden the water of the True One, once known as the Yin Tiger; and also, that 'a fluid is born from within the heart' and that within this fluid is hidden the vapour of the Proper Yang, once known as the Yang Dragon.

The Dragon and Tiger may also stand at times for the breath of the liver and lungs. This is truly the mystery of all mysteries. For if you understand how to foster and refine their separate breaths, you know also how to mix with the divine.

NOTE: The above section contains the essence of the chapter. It describes the Yin Tiger water and Yang Dragon vapour.

The collection of texts *Upon the Transmission of the Path* also states that the vapour of the kidneys is passed on to the breath of the heart and that it is their accumulated breaths that give birth to a fluid – whilst within this fluid lies the vapour of the Proper Yang, known as the Yang Dragon. This is also what is meant by 'emerging from out the fire'.

It also states that the fluid of the heart is passed on to the fluid of the kidneys and that it is their accumulated fluids that give birth to an energy – whilst within this energy lies the water of the True One, known as the 'Yin Tiger'. This is also what is meant by being 'born again out the water'.

On the occasion these two animals join, 'within the man, is born a man', that is, within each of us is born a spirit, living and quite divine.

Throughout all ages, this view of the Dragon and Tiger has perhaps involved too much cleverness and theorising. We know that the Dragon does not directly refer to the liver and the Tiger to the lungs, but how does one apprehend their 'moment of union' and awaken to their 'method of capture'? This may well be asked – because it is not uncommon that some people achieve a Life Everlasting and ascend to be immortals. The best of all of them are amongst us.

THE *WESTERN MOUNTAIN RECORDS* STATE THAT ONCE water and fire have passed over, as in *Already Over* (Hexagram 63),[1] the Dragon and Tiger join together – but work in different ways. The *Western Mountain* records state various opinions on this matter.

Hexagram 63 – Already Over

For instance, the kidney-breath is said to be conducted into the liver, the liver-breath thence being born; the remainder of the kidney Yin then enters the spleen, its breath passing out over into the liver to form the purest Yang. Within this breath lies the water of the True One, which reaches into the heart.

---

1   Also known as *All Complete, Once Succeeded*, etc.

Then the accumulated breaths generate a fluid, which, drop by drop, 'like a suspended pearl of dangling dew', returns to the lower field of the body, where it is altered – not following the water usually voided through the bladder.

If you make use of 'timing its firing', without a single mistake, you then smelt its energy and create a single living breath.

'Within the breath is born a breath', alive and pliant, and it happens in such a fashion that you form a land-based Divine Immortal. This is the Tiger crossing the path of the Dragon and the breaths of the heart and kidneys joining together. That is all.

Also when lowering the Fire, there are moments when you either increase or decrease it – for instance, there is the idea of 'extraction' and 'adding on' until the breaths of the heart and kidneys join. In the same way, this is the Dragon crossing the path of the Tiger.

Take the lower regions. Starting from the point of the tailbone, as the breath ascends on the left it becomes a Dragon; as it arises on the right it turns into a Tiger.

The breath follows the mid-backbone through the Double Gates and crossing over them, reaches a divide in the track at the mountains above where the vapour of the Yang Dragon enters the Inner Duct whilst the breath of the Yin Tiger enters the Heavenly Pond. 'To the left it turns, to the right it revolves' thirty-six times – then the true water falls down, like sweet dew entering the heart. This is 'the Dragon and Tiger crossing paths at the Upper Palace'.

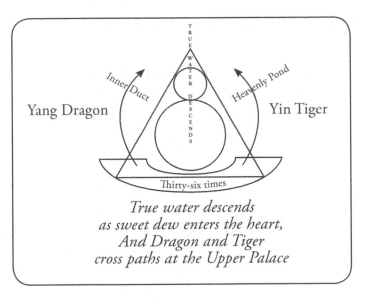

True water descends
as sweet dew enters the heart,
And Dragon and Tiger
cross paths at the Upper Palace

All Complete

This does not necessarily always involve the heart and kidneys, but it is another example of 'crossing and joining' – and also later on, once 'the foetus is finished and complete', the True Breath is born. To protect against this breath becoming over-full, you should try to aid it by using water, to create both the Jade Fluid and Golden Fluid Elixirs of Return.

NOTE: These ideas are further refinements of
the engagement of the Dragon and Tiger.

Another view is that as the Elixir of Return survives for a day, it travels along the channels and collaterals of the body and limbs, transforming into a Yang Cheese, which solidifies at the Central Palace (acupoint Lu.1), building into a substance not unlike white snow.

To protect against this substance becoming over-abundant, you should promote a fire, whence comes the 'smelting of matter and incineration of the self'. This is to understand the timing of the Elixir of Return, for if the Yin Tiger walks out singly, she will not engage with the Dragon – also then you can time the 'complete incineration of matter', for if the Yang Dragon rises alone, he will not engage with the Tiger.

> *NOTE: The role of the 'white snow' and dual*
> *husbandry of the Dragon and Tiger was later*
> *expounded upon in the 400-character poem by Zhang*
> *Boduan: 'white snow falling out of emptiness…' etc.*
> *For the Elixir of Return see the next chapter.*

This business of the Dragon and Tiger is highly significant! Those who fail to understand it cannot properly comprehend their own birthright. If you have knowledge of the emblems of the Dragon and Tiger, and are also aware of their moment of union, at the final attempt you will succeed in the art of capturing them and keeping them alive. Then over three hundred days you may crystallise them into an Inner Elixir and your destiny be made brilliantly clear.

Then you gain a life-term equal to that of the Universe!

18

药丹

The True Medicinal Elixir

The true Elixir is the same as the true Medicine…take
any breath, return it to its source and you have the
Elixir of Return…

THE HIGHEST AND FIRST RULING PRINCIPLE OF ALL
finds its beginning in the dust of this world, but is transmitted on
down to the Great and Supreme Path itself; being present in the image
of the fitting rise and fall of the strengths of Heaven and earth, and
the frequent arrivals and departures of the sun and moon. This truth is
quite clearly stated in *The Annals Recorded on the Vault of the Sky.*

> NOTE: *The external heavenly phenomena*
> *of the sun and moon are evidenced to give*
> *an example of the work of the Elixir.*

Once Master Guang Zheng instructed our Yellow Emperor in these
practices, the Emperor tried to keep to them, but for a long time he
saw few results. Even though he practised every day any number of
arts, the source and root of his practice was not firm or reliable.

Then in the fastness of the hills he took hold of the craft of 'inner
affairs'. His model was that of combining metals and minerals, and
matching them up. Thus he came across the idea of an Elixir.

The internal Medicinal Elixir is the true Medicine, for the external Medicinal Elixir is only able to cure disease, and bring you contentment – that is all it can achieve. In the short run, the internal Elixir lengthens your life, and delays old age, but in the long run, you can manage to transcend earthly matters to 'walk in the divine'.

At its beginning, the two breaths lie mated together and condensed at the lower belly, transforming the fluid-essences into Mercury, the Mercury into Coarse Sand, and the Coarse Sand into an Elixir. It is just the size of a crossbow pellet, its colour dark red like lacquer. The True Breath is born in just such a fashion, quite spontaneously.

'Consider the breath when refining the breath' and the breath and the mind will combine together and you enter on, into the way of the Path. The Path succeeded upon, you enter on, into the way of the divine; divinity implies greatness and this transforms you. There is nothing now that is unaffected! How could an external Elixir ever do this!

> NOTE: *Understand that the true Elixir is the same*
> *as the true inner Medicine – nothing should be*
> *sought beyond the confines of your own true self.*

A SAYING FROM THE *WESTERN MOUNTAIN RECORDS* states, 'if you take the Dragon and Tiger joined in matrimony, they form together into a Dark Pearl; and if you time their firing without a break, you will succeed in cooking the Great Medicine.'

> NOTE: *Here is outlined the whole picture of so-called*
> *'inner affairs'. First identify and separate out the materials,*
> *'dragon and tiger', 'lead and mercury', 'vapour and fluid',*
> *whatever; second combine and fire them, accordingly. By*
> *closely following the whole process, an Elixir will be created.*

As the True Breath is first born, then rising, it refines the physical body, so that then you no longer suffer from cold and heat. Once the True Breath is gathered and taken in, it restores the Elixir, so you permanently evade both hunger and thirst. If it can do all this, it must surely be some Medicine!

As the True Breath is displayed to others, it has similar results. Plunge it into water and the water boils; blow it against a plant and the plant springs into life; it turns pain into pleasure, and weakness to strength. If a man or woman uses it to relieve suffering, there is nothing they cannot heal – as it condenses into spirit it shakes out devils and goblins. Then there are none that do not miraculously respond.

The saying goes: 'If the inner is true, the outer must follow.' Thenceforth surely this must be a medicine for all!

But if 'inner affairs' are not taken care of, or the source is missed, and people only employ external and senseless metals and minerals, day after day they increase the heat, brew up and drink down the resulting mixture and think they will rise up again and be saved. How wrong they are!

However, it is also true that at all times the best scholars have also spoken of an external Elixir. It is not that it has never been used. For instance, Master Guang Zheng used 'red sand' as his elixir, refined it nine times and called it a 'holy medicine'; and the Seven-times Told Master seven times took his treasured 'elixial sand', refined it nine times and called it a 'miraculous medicine', whilst King Liu took young boys' fresh urine, refined it seven times, and named it an 'elixir of return'. They knew how to use this miraculous combining together of materials to form something magic and as this magic scattered they entered the Void, making their breath 'return to the source'. This is why it was called an 'elixir of return'. Later generations used these ideas and also saw the same result – and they rose above, to become immortals.

The first and only thing to do is to properly understand the processes of refinement, and the cycles of heating and cooling, so that 'inner affairs' as well as outer affairs may be taken care of. When internal and external both succeed together, you may then gain entrance to the Path of the Immortals.

But if you employ outer medicines alone, the breath weakens and the spirit is lost; you cannot retain the luxuriant breath of the skies and the earth and, on the contrary, great harm is done.

19

铅汞

The True Lead and Mercury

Lead represents the breath of the kidneys, Mercury
represents the heart's fluid…

IN ANCIENT TIMES, AS THE LAST CHAPTER RECORDED,
Old Master Zheng instructed the Yellow Emperor, who was intent
upon refining an outer Elixir. Then the Emperor hit upon the idea
of making an inner Elixir – and thenceforth came into being the use
of the materials 'lead' and 'mercury', the 'inner affairs' of the body
being fashioned and made use of through partaking in a model of the
outer, external world. This story is told also in *The Jade Summons on
the Dark Vault*.

For instance, when a human child is initially created, the first
organs to come into being are the kidneys. The kidneys reflect the
water of the Northern Realms, being associated with 'dark lead'
within the Five Metals; next to be created is the heart – the heart
reflects the fire of the Southern Realms, associating with 'coarse sand'
amongst the Eight Minerals.

> *NOTE: Explaining how 'lead' and 'mercury' come
> into being in the human foetus. 'Coarse sand' is a
> term often used for the sulphate of mercury.*

Heart
COURSE SAND
Fire of the Southern Realms

Water of the Northern Realms
DARK LEAD
Kidneys

Now when from this Lead is derived a silvery substance, it is like the darkly concealed water of the True One hidden in the breath of the kidneys; whilst when from Coarse Sand you can derive Mercury, it is like the darkly concealed vapour of the Proper Yang hidden within the breath of the heart.

Now in the outer world, if you take the 'silver within lead' and mix it with the 'mercury of the coarse sand', the mixture becomes all sand; and when the firing is timed appropriately, you will finally refine and complete a great treasure.

If you apply this process to the human body, then the water of the True One is derived from the breath of the kidneys, and the vapour of the Proper Yang derived from the heart's fluid. These two materials join together to form a Medicinal Elixir.

And this is similar in comparison to any visible treasure that we can create in the outer material world.

> *NOTE: Lead, from being dark, turns silvery and becomes
> fluid, when heated. This is used as an image of the 'water
> hidden within the kidneys'. Mercuric sulphate or 'coarse
> sand' releases its mercury, also when heated. This is used*

as an analogy for the 'Yang hidden in the heart'. Thus
we are creating a precious treasure within the body.

THE *WESTERN MOUNTAIN RECORDS* STATE THAT THE
Anthology of the Transmission of the Tao from Zhong to Lu mentions
'cherishing the substance of heavenly unity, the True One', and it
promotes the first of the Five Metals, the Black Lead. Lead then gives
birth to silver. Lead is mother to silver.

Through the influence of the Greater Yang breath, the main of
the minerals, the 'red sand', is formed. Coarse Sand gives birth to
Mercury, whilst Mercury is child to the Red Sand.

It is difficult to extract the silvery substance derived from Lead,
and it is easy to lose the Mercury inhabiting the Red Sand. But if
Lead and Mercury can bond together and be smelted continuously, a
treasure will be rapidly formed.

NOTE: These external, physical minerals, Lead and Mercury,
illustrate a pattern that also happens in the inner world.

Now in terms of how things work inside the body, the True Breath
of our loving father and mother join together to form one – that is,
blood and essences make up the foetus in the womb. They consolidate
together, lining the kidneys, which implies they fashion the Lead of
the kidneys. So when a breath is born within the kidneys, within this
breath is born the kidney-water. You take the kidney-water to join
with the heart's fluid above, to form the vapour of the Proper Yang,
and then they consolidate at the Yellow Courtyard, creating an Elixir
– this implies that it must be the True Lead.

As the breaths of the kidneys and heart join, their amassed force
generates a fluid that congeals into a Dark Pearl. This means that again
it returns to the lower belly, and may be termed Mercury. Then once
this Elixir is finished it takes the True Breath up above – the breath
of the kidneys – to enter the crown of the head, whilst the true water
descends down below. The one rises, the other falls, in front of the

Twelve-Tiered Pagoda, and the process is named *Perfection*.[1] As soon as perfection is achieved, it returns again to the lower *dantian* – this implies that it must be the True Mercury.

Hexagram 63 – Perfection

The poem 'Lord of the Originating Imperial' goes:

> Flamed up to form a Peerless Pearl!
> All these Simple Folk arriving,
> Bring a knowledge of the Book of every School!

The True Master 'Proper Unity' says:

> Lead and Mercury have travelled Ten Thousand Autumns.
> How many people have awaken?
> How many people have tried?
> Suppose this Rule is taught
> To perpetuate human understanding,
> This Dusty World and the Holy Immortals
> Are all alike in one flowing Stream!

Duke Lu has said:

> A Single Grain of Golden Elixir
> Will give you Life Everlasting.
> You should acquire some True Lead
> And then fire it, first and last.
> The Fire caught in the Southern Realms
> Is the Red Phoenix's Marrow!
> The Water sought in the Northern Seas,
> The Black Tortoise's Seed!

---

1   Hexagram 63, also known as *Once Succeeded, All Complete, Already Over.*

Throughout the ages, the highest Sages have spoken of the 'lead' and 'mercury', but they never agreed completely upon what they meant by them.

They agree only on this: that the Lead represents the breath of the kidneys and that the True Lead fashions the Elixir, whilst the Mercury represents the heart's fluid and that the True Mercury fashions the medicine, and that the True Lead and Mercury mixed together form a happening that may be named *Perfection* (Hexagram 63), that is, one of 'mutual support'.

Take a more literal view and you will forfeit the inner Path!

20

阳 阳

The True Yin and Yang

> ...if you quieten the breath ten thousand times, the
> worldly breath will depart, the spirit be conserved,
> and the result be the creation of a Great Vehicle of
> Enlightenment.

ONE YIN AND ONE YANG SIGNIFY THE PATH, AND WHEN
Yin and Yang are unfathomable, they signify the spirit. This is stated
in *The Secret Registry on the Nine Heavens.*

Contained within all things lies our spiritual Majesty. Heaven
acquires the single Yang and thereby protects the Path of the trigram
Qian ☰; the earth acquires the single Yin and thus protects the Path
of the trigram Kun ☷.

Contained within all things, there also lies a spiritual brilliance.
The sun acquires the single Yang, the Hun-soul, and thus the Path is
brought to our notice; the moon acquires the single Yin, the Po-soul,
and thus the Path is finally attained.

> *NOTE: The single Yin and single Yang, the sun and*
> *moon, Hun and Po-souls; the Path brought to our notice,*
> *the Path attained. The opening words to this chapter*
> *derive from the Great Appendix (Xici) to the Yijing.*

At the summer solstice, the single Yin of winter arrives from the
heavens and if there were no True Yang, all things would perish

through the Winter Yin and not be able to be unfolded by the gentle warmth of spring; at the winter solstice the single Yang of summer appears from the earth and if there were no True Yin, all things would be born from the Yang, but not be able to be nourished through the Yin moisture of autumn.

> *NOTE: The interdependence of Yin and Yang is illustrated in the idea of the passing seasons, which nourish all life on earth. The gentle heat of the spring is needed – as is the True Yang – to prevent all things perishing through the Winter Yin cold. The cooling dews of autumn likewise enable the nourishment of the True Yin; otherwise we would all perish in the heat of the Summer Yang.*

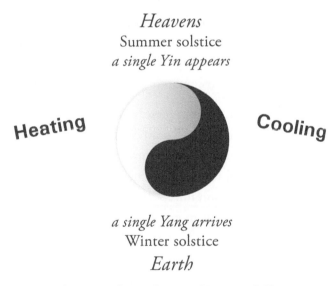

Heavens
Summer solstice
a single Yin appears

Heating   **Cooling**

a single Yang arrives
Winter solstice
Earth

The Interdependence of Yin and Yang

The sun represents the presence of the True Yang – for when the Focusing Mirror catches the sun's rays during the day, a spark of fire is born; furthermore, the moon reveals the absence of the True Yin – for when the 'Watery Toad' (a kind of condensing pot) catches the moon's rays at night, a watery fluid condenses. Thus is displayed the ultimate majesty and brilliance of Heaven and earth, the sun and moon. You need look no further than at these kind for the True Yin and True Yang!

THE SAGES OF THE WESTERN MOUNTAIN ARE RECORDED as stating that the kidneys represent the element water. Whilst within this water is born the vapour of the true fire and within this breath is hidden the 'water of the True One'. This is the Yang within the Yin, and the Yin within the Yang.

Likewise the heart represents the element fire. Whilst within this fire is produced the fluid of the true water, and within this fluid is hidden the 'vapour of the Proper Yang'. This is the Yin within the Yang, and the Yang within the Yin.

There are three glories, because there are Three Yang: the breath of the kidneys is the Yang within the Yin; the True Breath settled within the Elixir is the Yang within the True Yang; and the breath of the heart's fluid is the Yang within the Yang. The Three Yin are not discussed, because to value the Yin is to contaminate the purity of the Yang.

According to the ancient writings preserved within the *Rhymes on the Jade and August Holy Foetus*, we should constantly sink the heart-fire down into the Lower Field (*dantian*, lower belly). Do not let outer influences affect you and utterly eradicate any wild imaginings, that the Single Breath may remain unbroken.

Abandon yourself totally to the 'sea of the breathing', that the breath beneath the kidneys may be encouraged not to rise up; as the breath gradually lessens, in a relaxed manner, you may let the True Breath emerge. Then all thoughts and worries will ebb away. This results in what the latter Sages identified as the spontaneous 'foetal breath'.

Yang within the Yin,
Yin within the Yang

FIRE

Fluid of the True Water
Breath of the Proper Yang

◯

Water of the True One
Breath of the True Fire

WATER

Yin within the Yang,
Yang within the Yin

Again, Bodhidharma in his *Supreme Method of the Foetal Breath* stated, 'if we allow our breath to rise upwards, we are lost.' There is no better practice, in his view, than the 'inner gazing' of the several worlds, that we may amuse ourselves playing in the Hall of Heaven, and escape into the clear void and Place of All Mysteries.

His practice especially paid attention to 'not leaking' – when 'no single thought was allowed to arise, no single idea to be born'.

Through 'not leaking' he attained the very best of results, and, undisturbed, was able to find a firm regard for the true divine. He remained sitting 'with his face to the wall nine years'. He allowed not the slightest breath to escape and all the dark forces ranged against him scattered, of their own accord.

Thus 'without his body, he found a body'. But as the people of the Eastern world did not understand this method, he threw away his begging-bowl and returned to the West. After some time had passed, the Sages called this practice the true 'foetal breath'.

> *NOTES: The legend is of this Chan monk's interview with the Emperor, where Bodhidharma was disgusted by the Emperor's lack of perception. This story is well known.*

It is just as Bian Que, in his commentary on the *Spiritual Pivot*, described. When it came to the time just after the winter solstice, when a fraction of the True Lead accumulates within the body, shaped like a 'sporting stamen', then he crushed it down into his *dantian*. He instructed his people to use the nose to guide in the clean air, to close up the mouth and not let the breath out, settling the breath twenty-four times to build up a single ounce of Fire – after which, in forty-five days, the Fire builds to sixteen ounces and he would have completed the Yang Foetus.

Accordingly, at the time after the summer solstice, when a 'small egg of Yin' accumulates within the body, he crushed it down into the Lower Palace. He instructed his people to use the nose to guide in the clean air, to close up the mouth and not let it out, settling the breath twenty-four times to build a single ounce of Fire – after which, in forty-five days, the Fire builds to sixteen ounces, and he would have refined the Yin Breath.

Taking the Yin Breath, cast it into the Yang Foetus and you give birth to the True Breath. Then the True Breath gives birth to the Source Spirit, the spiritual and physical merge, and with Heaven and earth you may end your days. Yet split them apart and they remain as two: for 'without the body there is a body'.

This enables you to be a lighter-than-air guest at the gathering of the Immortals. You no longer remain in this dusty world, but retire to the Three Isles and Ten Islets, adrift on a broad ocean.

> *NOTE: Bian Que was the legendary physician who lived around the fourth century BCE.*

As Ge Hong commented in his *Discourse on the Foetal Breath*, 'generally the foetal breath has one crucial distinction; it is as if you were still held in your mother's belly.'

> As your mother breathes out,
> So you breathe out.
> As your mother breathes in,
> So you breathe in.

The present population does not apprehend this Method of All Mysteries. Although they are able to close off their breath in an instant, they soon lose interest, and the rough breath never comes to an end. Not only are they unable to retain the closure of the breath, but furthermore the source breath itself declines and naturally weakens. Then their worldly breath appears outward and their strength is wasted.

If the breath starts to speed up, then before it becomes too rapid, cause it to be held outside the body a short while – without forcing it. At the exact moment, just before it accelerates, let the nose guide in a mouthful of clean air, continuously exchanging the newly acquired breath for the old, transforming the remainder of the breath. In such a fashion you can steal upon the departure of the worldly breath.

As this process builds up, the mind and body will become clear and enlivened, and you are able to expel and cure any disease. But beware! To stiffen yourself in keeping up this practice and to force the departure of the worldly breath is unnatural. This is simply 'lower-order foetal breathing'.

The True Immortals and honoured Sages developed a Theory of Three Categories. To guide the breath through the nose and expel the worldly breath through the mouth can dispel a superficial cold, chase away residual fevers, shake up knotty blockages, and even enliven the channels and collaterals. This is the *first* category of the breath.

But as you quieten the breath, the breath and the blood become engaged. Then Yin and Yang are tangled in intercourse. This is the *second* category of the breath.

Once you have settled the breath ten thousand times, the breath departs and the spirit congeals. This is the Great Vehicle; but of this I cannot speak. This is the *third* category of the breath. Of all methods of fortifying the breath, this is the best.

Perhaps you swallow down the breath to help hunger or thirst, or direct it to strengthen the flesh and muscles, or draw it in to build up the Lower Field (*dantian*), or sustain it in order to regain a youthful complexion. This is to circulate around the worldly breath, which benefits the blood vessels, but it sees only minor improvements.

In the last analysis, if you do not apply the power of the foetal breath which rebuilds the worldly breath, and through which you gain inner strength, where are you? The merit of your work is speedily gone…

The Refinement

21

Refining the Method, You Walk the Path

A student of the Path should find no obstacles; if you
find any obstacles, your Method is untrue.

THE *WESTERN MOUNTAIN RECORDS* STATE THAT IF YOU
use the method of sustaining the breath to approach the Path, the
Path will present no impossibilities, whilst if you use the Path to seek
immortality, immortality becomes simple.

When seeking immortality, there should be no obstacles; if you
find any obstacles in your Path, it is because your Path is incorrect.

A student of the Path should find no obstacles; if he finds any
obstacles in the method, it is because his method is untrue.

*NOTE: This is how to refine a method to walk the
Path. The method referred to in this chapter is the Way
of Yin and Yang. The best is to be 'free and easy'.*

The ancient peoples 'hid their traces, changed their appearances',
'retained their breath to return the Hun-soul', 'muttered oaths over a
naked sword blade', restrained poisonous insects from biting, bound
themselves severely with ties, trod on fire without being burnt, caused
water to flow backward, drummed up the wind and rain, threw a

cloth on the ground and caught rabbits, entangled and deceived snakes, caused the instant ripening of melons and fruits, and so on and so forth.

All such tricks as these are clever arts, but they have nothing to do with the method of walking on the Path!

And again when the Yang was born at the end of winter, after the spring equinox, when a remnant of cold was plaguing the stomach and intestine, and presenting as a cold-injury, once the ancients saw this, they rapidly:

> Hid themselves away in an uncluttered room,
> Crossed the legs and sat upright,
> Closed the eyes and dimmed the heart,
> Settling the breath to expel worldly stuffs.

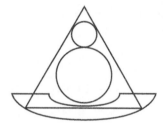 Then with both hands folded on top of one another, they scoured the area around the loins, until, in no more than twenty or thirty measures, a clear sweat came out along with the chill, and the cold vapour scattered of its own accord.

And when they had 'dream-cast sperm' at night-time, if the lower belly was weak and cold, at the end of the day, they would 'sit up still, in a darkened room, using the hands to scour the area around the loins, using the hands to chafe beneath the navel eighty-one times, chafing the hands and rubbing the loins, scouring with the hands and chafing the navel area eighty-one times, nine rounds, one measure; left and right exchanging hands' and then finish.

In this fashion the elixial belly recovered its warmth, and the True Breath was filled and replete.

The ancient peoples used:

> A silent retreat in a quiet room,
> Ceased all thinking and forgot all speech,

Wholly directing the fire down beneath,
Closed the eyes and preserved their ideas...

Until like a wheel of fire, flickering and glowing, their breath accumulated daily at the 'sea of the breath' (lower belly), solid and strong, and their complexion changed constantly. Day after day they practised, until, over several seasons, they were able to naturally bear both heat and cold.

And when their dietary habits got out of hand and the belly and gut were overfull, or else a fever was blocked up within, or painful knots and aches obstructed the limbs and channels, then...

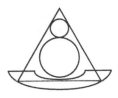

They sat up quietly,
The nose guiding in the clear breath,
The mouth shut and unopened,
'Taking in more, letting out less'
To attack the area of the disease.

If there were complications, then they let the breath go, but not less than four or five times, so that naturally any troubles ebbed and eased; and over a long period of time they got rid of every single disease.

And also when their limbs had any small ailment or else the internal organs were slightly ill, either through being blocked, or obstructed...

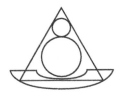

They sat quietly, clearly, purely,
Closed the eyes, and ceased all thinking.

In such a manner, they directed the breath to the exact site of the disease and briefly retained it there a short while.

Using these methods, there is nothing in this world you cannot touch and alter. There is nothing you cannot conquer. However, the above techniques are indeed all 'methods', but they have nothing to do with the Path!

As for the Path, there is nothing it does not embrace, there is nowhere it cannot reach. How can it consist only in such clever tricks, and healing disease, and that be all!

But follow these arts and you will understand about methods, and follow the methods and you will understand about the Path.

The Path is fundamentally one single Yin and one single Yang. And that is that.

> NOTE: *The Dao or Path is 'one Yin and Yang and this is all'. This statement comes from the Great Appendix (Xici) to the Yijing. It sets the seal on a characteristically Chinese approach to immortality – the Dao cannot be limited to any one thing beyond Yin and Yang.*

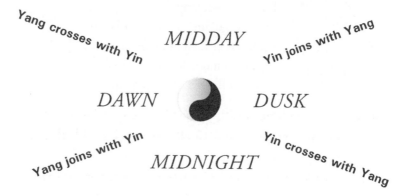

True Yin and Yang, Born in the Outside World

AS YIN AND YANG JOIN AND CROSS, THEY CAUSE HEAVEN and earth to create the four seasons of spring, summer, autumn and winter, just as the sun and moon present the four periods of waxing, full, waning and new moon. And so it is within man, during each day and night:

> At the end of the period after midnight
> And the start of the period before dawn,
> The Yang joins with the Yin;
> At the end of the period of early morning
> And the beginning of period of mid-morn,
> The Yang crosses with the Yang;

At the end of the period just after midday
And the start of the period of the afternoon,
The Yin joins with the Yang;
And at the end of the period of early even'
And the start of the period of late evening,
The Yin crosses with the Yin.

Understand the 'joining and crossing' of Yin and Yang, and you cannot be far from the Path!

22

化

Refining the Body,
You Transform the Breath

> ...allow the breath through the nose to enter in a little
> and then slowly, slowly to come out, like a thread of
> silken twine, scarcely held...until you can refine the
> breath and fashion the spirit.

THE *WESTERN MOUNTAIN RECORDS* STATE THAT THE
breath inhabits the body whilst the breath is the commander of the
body. As the body sustains the breath, the breath becomes robust
and the body truly strong; as the breath is circulated around the
body it itself becomes refined, the body whole and the breath gains
the merit of the True Breath. This is a truth stated in the *Western
Mountain Records*.

The Great Circulation of the True Breath of each individual
follows the timing of the heavens.

> In spring it has to do with the liver,
> In summer it has to do with the heart,
> In autumn it inhabits the lungs,
> In winter it lives in the kidneys.

As for man's Silent Breath, its Small Circulation follows the times of the day: at midnight it has to do with the kidneys, at dawn with the liver, at midday with the heart, at dusk with the lungs.

> *NOTE: These are not necessarily the actual dawn, midday, dusk and midnight. They are the 'living dawn', 'living midday', etc. They can occur at any time and are not specific to any particular hour. It is up to us to be aware.*

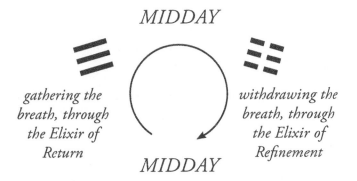

In ancient times the intelligent people of this world knew how to lay bare the Workings of Heaven: they took the measure of man's breath to be one with the heavens and took its daily function and combined it with its yearly function.

From midnight to midday, as the breath is born, they used the method of 'gathering the breath' through the Elixir of Return, whilst from midday to midnight, as the breath dispersed, they used the method of 'withdrawing the breath' through the Elixir of Refinement.

> *NOTE: Thus first comes the birth, the gathering power of the breath of Qian-heaven, the father, the dragon; next comes the refinement, the withdrawing power of Kun-earth, the mother, the mare. These images are all taken from the Yijing. Adept Jade Peng's song goes: 'In the morning train up the Dragon! After midday train up the Mare!'*

From early dawn onwards to midday raise up the body, quietly sitting still, dim the sight and forget all speech, the breath coming in through the nose slower and slower...

Then you can confine your thoughts to the Heart Palace, and your ideas appear as 'husband and wife in each other's loving embrace'. After a long, long period of time the task will be complete, and you succeed in achieving Life Everlasting, an existence beyond death.

In ancient times the elderly adept Breaking Bright Dawn's song went:

> In the morning I get up without a word,
> Take the tongue and stir under the top palate,
> Beneath it turbid juices are spat out.

This is to expel the emotions of joy, anger, sadness and pleasure, which all have their accumulation within the heart. The True Breath will then rise upwards, lingering and retained at the 'face and eyes' – where you may make use of every intention to grasp hold of it.

Next he made a space in a quiet room, sitting peacefully without speaking until the interval just before midday. The breath filled out and his mind dimmed. Then he lay down on his side, closed his lips gently, and slept.

Over many days he peaceably and joyfully delayed the onset of old age, retained his physical body and departed this dusty world. Thus he was able to comprehend the idea of 'term and hour', to awaken to the phrase 'joining and crossing', and this was all achieved without any method of capturing or extracting a medicine. Indeed he was a clever fellow.

THE SAGES OF THE WESTERN MOUNTAIN UNDERSTOOD that at the instant of midnight the kidney-breath comes alive, at dawn the liver-breath comes alive, whilst at midday the kidney-breath joins with that of the heart and their accumulated breaths generate a fluid, which – returned to the *dantian* – may be termed a 'dark pearl'.

If the firing is then timed without interruption, you can complete a supreme Medicine.

Within the kidney-breath is hidden the water of the True One, whilst along with the heart's fluid is hidden the vapour of the Proper Yang. Take Yin to embrace Yang, and you make use of the liquid fluid to absorb an energy – which is the root of the Great Path, the Medicine of Life Everlasting! How can we then employ this medicine, so as not to lose it?

> *NOTE: The above practice describes 'gathering the breath'*
> *through the Elixir of Return. From midnight up to midday,*
> *Yin is embracing Yang. How to employ it so as not to lose it?*
> *The answer is given below. The timing is only suggestive.*

During the time between early and late morning, in a darkened room sit up quietly, the mind and understanding held within, the mouth gathered full of saliva – do not swallow it, do not spit it out; then allow the breath to run in through the nose, a little at a time, and then slowly, slowly to run out – until it appears to exist as a continuous silken thread, barely held in the hand.

Then of their own accord the two breaths will combine, condensing like settling dew. Practise this method one hundred days without interruption and the power of the Medicine is complete; two hundred days and the Holy Foetus is strong; three hundred days and a Foetal Immortal is grown. Thus is the True Breath born.

Then 'within the breath there is a breath', and you are next able to refine the breath to 'fashion the spirit', as described in the following chapter.

Mr Zhong Li comments: Of old there have been just a few truths – and only a few rhymes commending the True Golden Elixir. If you are not aware of these truths in your practice, your worldly study of the Path is ill-spent and a wearisome task.

He goes on to state:

> Leisurely and unoccupied
> The river flows to the South,
> The flowers blooming
> Full in the spring pastures,

The waters limpid…
If you see the one you love,
You have an inclination to pole secretly out…
About on the Tiger and Dragon bateau.

This is called the 'Dragon and Tiger courting together', and again, it is the method by which you may pluck a Medicinal Herb from which to create an Elixir.

> *NOTE: When 'within the breath there is a breath' you are next able to refine this breath to 'fashion the spirit'. This is described in the next chapter. Here we enter the morning experience of the Medicinal Herb. We are transported by the doting affection between Yin and Yang. The southern direction is the direction of Fire. In the spring fields, all the flowers come alive. Being infused with these 'animal passions' it is like going out to meet the one you love – you pole out on the flat waters, drifting to a secret tryst together. Truly this is the nub of the Method.*

On the methods of 'from midday to midnight, using the method of withdrawing the breath to smelt the Elixir', which describe the 'timing of the firing', people have not always agreed. But if you do not understand its true principle, you will not understand the Workings of Heaven. Then how are you fit to reach into the Treasure Chest of Creation! Only Bian Que understood and communicated it to us in the *Lingshu* medical classic, saying… 'use the nose to take in the clean breath, and as it enters then retain it slightly, four breaths and you make one grain, twenty-four grains and you make a single ounce of fire.'

After the summer has arrived, take the Sun-wind trigram 'at the twenty-fifth measure of the round of the Heavenly Dew' and practise it, and smelt the True Mercury to create a Yin Foetus; and when the winter arrives take the Qian-heaven trigram 'at the twenty-fifth measure of the round of the Spiritual Token' and practise it, and smelt the True Lead to create the Yang Breath. The Yang finished, the Yin Foetus may be cast aside, and it changes into a Golden Elixir – one grain of this Elixir can give you long life, and after this you never perish.

Master Guang Zheng taught the Yellow Emperor, from dawn to dusk, to 'sit quietly, forgetting all thought', screening off all intercourse with outer ideas, his mind and understanding held within, a single intent undivided; he instructed him to sink his heart-fire into the lower belly, caring for the area beneath the navel to make it like a washed-out jar. Within this washed-out jar, there then came into being a pearl the shape of a crossbow pellet.

Take this blazing fire, day or night, and get to work on firing the pearl and the Foetus is complete with the common breath departed. Then you naturally feel neither hunger nor thirst, nor dread the winter-cold nor feel the summer-heat. You are able both to retain your physical body and depart this dusty world.

> *NOTE: This paragraph describes how to gain the ability,*
> *dawn to dusk, of advancing the firing of an Elixir.*

THE PEOPLE OF WESTERN MOUNTAIN HAVE A HYMN that goes:

> When a beautiful lad and lass
> Find the right moment,
> Rich fall the blooms in the soft twilight…
> If they do not hesitate to interrupt
> Their chief desire,
> Presently they find a way to the Yang Gate!

This illustrates how, halfway through the evening, the breath follows the opportunity created by the True Fluid Elixir of Return – now the Yin is joining with more Yin and its breath is at the point of being dispersed and lost.

At this moment you should make some space in a quiet room, the breath not closed off, but only a little taken in – and slowly let out; then lower the heart-fire down, until the mind is retained at the lower belly. Be careful, lest the breath of the kidneys rise up without stopping. Let the heart-fire only be lowered down and not depart. This is to gently use a little force lightly applied to the tummy and abdomen, until the *dantian* becomes warm of its own accord.

> *NOTE: In the above poem, the boy and girl represent*
> *Yang and Yin. At the right moment the rich bloom of*
> *the spirit imbues the twilight hour. Only be careful.*
> *Do not harbour too much want, but neither interrupt*
> *your chief desire and you will find your way to the*
> *Portals of Heaven, the Yang Gate. This is the 'evening*
> *procedure' of withdrawing and conserving the breath.*

As you enter these days of refinement, during which you also obtain the Medicine, the first hundred days you feel the strength of the Qian-heaven trigram; the next hundred days the attraction of the Dui-marsh trigram along with the great Qian trigram; the next hundred days the gentleness of the Kun-earth trigram along with the great Qian trigram. Now Qian and Kun are like 'husband and wife in each other's embrace', and the 'timing of their firing' goes uninterrupted.

In such a manner do 'increase and decrease unite accordingly', akin to the idea of 'extract and augment' – and there should 'immediately appear on hand a staggering golden hue'.

Anciently the Former High Sages spoke about this moment in the same fashion. They captured the medicine at the trigram of the brilliant Li-fire; they advanced the fire at the strong Qian-heaven. Three hundred days later they had again formed fully an Inner Elixir and became land-based Divine Immortals.

The body and spirit together are ultimately altogether marvellous! They are wholly living, pliable and undying. Follow the above procedures of refining the body and you will well understand how the Path lies totally within an acquired knowledge of the True Breath.

> *NOTE: This lovely section describes the true ease of Yin*
> *and Yang, the Tiger and Dragon bateau; the sense of*
> *the boat going of its own accord, just flowing, drifting*

along on its mission, quite hidden from the mortal world – the breath just moving on, naturally.

23

神

With a Refined Breath, You Can Fashion the Spirit

...in a quiet room sweep away all thoughts, and shut the eyes, sitting upright wrapped in oneself; then the breath of its own accord gathers, gently, gently, slowly, slowly, ascending the body...

THE *WESTERN MOUNTAIN RECORDS* STATE THAT YOU take the breath in order to refine the body. Once the body is transformed by the breath, your whole self will become light and nimble. You may enter water without drowning, and walk on fire and not get burnt. This is indeed stated in the *Western Mountain Records*.

What is of supreme importance is to marry together the Dragon and Tiger, in the manner described in the few last chapters, and thus fashion a Great and Holy Medicine. If the 'timing of the firing' is watched over faultlessly, the Medicine will then transform gradually into a Golden Elixir.

Immediately there appears on hand a Staggering Hue...
From behind at Tailgate Village
It ascends along the Central Spine;

From the Central Spine through Two Gates,
It ascends until it reaches the Upper Palace.

Now not only do you use the kidney-breath to benefit the brain, but also, after midday, you lower down the true fire in order to refine the Elixir – finally obliterating the Yin shadow that the Yang may become perfectly clear.

For instance, at the hour of midnight, just as the breath of the kidneys is born, in a quiet room sweep away all thought from the heart, and shut the eyes, sitting upright, wrapped in one's self – and the kidney-breath will, of its own accord, gather together, gently, gently, slowly, slowly ascending the body, through the chest, the waist, reaching the Central Spine and then the Upper Palace.

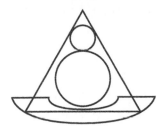

From midnight it builds up until early morn to mid-morning.

Settle this one hundred days, and it strikes against the Three Gates. Then again the true fire of the heart accumulates, forging and smelting an Inner Elixir at the Lower Source; the Yin solid and the Yang condensed, the breath of its own accord ravelled in confusion. This is known as 'the breath within the breath'.

In front it ascends into the crown of the head, whilst behind it rises to enter the brain. As front and behind rise together, they only ascend through the body – they do not disturb it – until finally they incinerate every single part of it, evicting all shady Yin devils.

One blaze adds on one breath; ten blazes add on one spirit; a hundred blazes lengthen our life ten thousand years; a thousand blazes and we exit this dusty world.

NOTE: Tailgate Village may be acupoint Du.2.
You take on the breath in order to refine the body.
This is all described in the previous chapter.

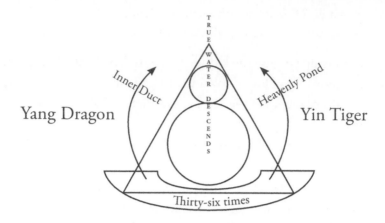

THE ANCIENT SAGES OF OLD WERE FEARFUL LEST THE Fire grew to excess; therefore they also derived the rule of 'washing and bathing' the Medicine.

At first, when secured, it is the Jaden Fluid Elixir of Return; 'immediately it appears on hand as a staggering hue' entering the brain. Then from the Upper Field, it should be returned to the Lower Field. This is the Rule of the Golden Fluid Elixir of Return. Take the cheeks and bulge them out, weakly blowing the breath out and in; this is all you need do. The Elixir complete, the True Breath is born – now you may use the True Breath to further refine the breath of the Five Treasury Organs.

> NOTE: *This is also described in detail in*
> *Chapter 16 on The True Water and Fire.*

The Book of the Nine Immortals states: To refine the Holy Sword and Golden Bludgeon, first use the breath of the Five Treasuries.

The Book of the Central Yellow Kingdom states: To close up the mouth through a thousand breaths is to refine the Five Treasuries.

The Sages of the Western Mountain have a Rule in refining the breath that is subtly and secretly preserved.

Capture the Medicine and advance the firing,
Three hundred days the Medicine is complete;
Return the Elixir to refine the Body,
Two hundred days the True Breath is filled.

For this method it is not necessary to follow the Great Circulation of Heaven through the seasons; you need only use the Small Circulation corresponding to the cycle of the days. Simply close up the breath and refine it.

For example, on liver-wood days you should refine the liver-breath. On the first day the liver-breath advances in the Gen-mountain trigram, seal it up until the time of the Sun-wind – it is like a Green Vapour seen, circulating around and reaching to the crown. On the second day sustain its breath, the same as the method above. In general as you begin 'timing its firing', you understand the mutually giving birth and conquest Cycles of the Five Powers.

On heart-fire days you should refine the heart-breath. On the first day the heart-breath advances in the Sun-wind trigram, seal off its breath until the time of the Kun trigram – it is like a Red Vapour seen, circulating around and reaching to the crown. On the second day sustain its breath. In general as you begin 'timing its firing', you understand the mutually giving birth and conquest Cycles of the Five Powers.

On spleen-earth days, you should refine the spleen-breath. As it first advances, fresh and eager, at early morning for a single hour, seal off its breath; in summer then just after midday seal off its breath; in the autumn in the early evening seal off its breath; in winter after midnight seal off its breath. In general as you begin 'timing its firing', you understand the mutually giving birth and conquest Cycles of the Five Powers.

On lung-metal days, you should refine the lung-breath. The first day the lung-breath advances in the Kun-earth trigram, seal off its breath until the time of the Qian-heaven trigram – it is like a White Vapour seen, circulating around and reaching to the crown. On the second day sustain its breath. In general as you begin 'timing its firing', you understand the mutually giving birth and conquest Cycles of the Five Powers.

On kidney-water days, you should refine the breath of the kidneys. The first day the breath of the kidneys advances in the Qian trigram, seal off its breath, until the time of the Gen-mountain trigram – it is like a Black Vapour seen, circulating around and reaching to the crown. On the second day sustain its breath. In general as you begin 'timing its firing', you understand the mutually giving birth and conquest Cycles of the Five Powers.

Now in ten days, through the Ten Heavenly Stems, you come back to refining a round of the Five Organs, so that in two hundred and fifty days, each is refined twenty-five times. Then the True Breath gathers of its own accord, starting off the Chain-and-Bucket Water Pump that transports up the substance of the Five Splendid Colours. It is:

> Like a group of girls playing on hand-held,
>   blown reed-organs,
> Horses with carriages, banners and fluttering flags,
> Each divided into its destined company and file,
> Assembled above at the Celestial Portal,
> Entering in together, on high, at the Heavenly Gate!

If perhaps Yin devils create obstacles, or evil spooks make difficulties for you, then only enter into a quiet room, close up the eyes and dim the heart, raise up the body and sit up straight.

Then give them a taste of the true fire, which comes alive of its own accord! A single blaze – and the spooks and devils ebb away. As the fire crosses over, you are washed clean and cool, your mind distinct and clear, whilst 'before you await several followers, singing and playing, clustered and gathered together full'.

Then all day you can sit quietly silently, your 'inner view' clear and intelligent, without ever having enough; enduring, wonderful sights and experiences are seen, evidencing different signs, which can never ever be totally described or written down.

Once you are aware of this, the physical body and form constantly resemble a flying phoenix. The mind and breath scoot around the body and can be difficult to rein in or control – so constantly make use of the harmonised mind, by refining the spirit to 'exit the husk', as described in the next chapter.

Then you may take the opportunity to transcend earthly matters and 'walk in the divine'.

> *NOTE: Notice the ecstatic and mystical state of the blended*
> *Five Splendid Colours, transported upwards, which*
> *evidences the spirit. The noise and grandeur of a group of*
> *girls blowing on musical hand-held reed organs (or sheng)*
> *is very pleasant…together they enter along with us into a*
> *'Celestial Portal' and through a 'Heavenly Gate'. It has been*
> *the same throughout all ages and cultures of humankind.*

24

With a Refined Spirit, You Can Join on the Path

...within your body 'clustered flowers' untangle, you return to cast your eyes on the Old Orchard...a solitary village-home!

THE *WESTERN MOUNTAIN RECORDS* STATE THAT THE fellow who cultivates the truth sets his mind on the Silent Source and on achieving sweet solitude. One day his breath fills out, and his work is complete – 'the Five Vapours assemble at the first gate, Three Flowers clustered at the crown'. The blood condenses, the breath gathers in, and a myriad beings are assembled there in truth. This is a truth asserted by the *Western Mountain Records*.

> At this exact moment
> You abide at the Upper Palace,
> Riches and honours arrive in abundance:
> A many-storied terrace
> Thronged with horses and carriages,
> Men and women mingled together
> As thickly as blown reeds
> On a hand-held reed-organ.

But even these folk are people of the ordinary world, the mortal world: this is not to gain complete recognition of your true condition. It is your body's Upper Palace, but you have not yet shed the Inner Courtyard.

You can accompany and follow them along but you have not yet 'shed the husk', which is to be still trapped on the Dark Thoroughfare of a mortal life.

NOTE: This poem expresses the bliss of transcendence. Note on how to 'shed the husk' or escape the wheel of transmigration.

As it has been said, the body and spirit are altogether mysterious! If you can never transcend them, you only become a land-based Divine Immortal. It is difficult then to 'shed your husk' and return to the Ten Islets and Three Holy Isles of the Immortals.

Before the work of the Ancient Sages of Western Mountain drew to a close, they achieved a method of 'shedding the husk', but were never able to write it down in detail.

But it is told that once upon a time, when Old Master Sea Toad's task was complete and his life's work fulfilled, he was at rest within his Upper Palace, the Yang on the point of 'shedding his husk'. Then he went to his room, to sit quietly in solitary silence. All at once, like a crane flying out into the open sky, like a dragon returning to its lair, his Yang spirit furiously struck against the sky, until, of its own accord, the sky opened, he 'shed his husk' and was gone.

Mr Zhong Li, his life's work complete and task fulfilled, sat quietly and 'gazed within', just as you might surmount a Seven-Storied Jewelled Pagoda, from below to above, one step at a time, reaching each level without hurrying, but hankering after his body he never 'shed his husk' and remained a land-based Divine Immortal.

This was because, when his ascent was finished, he closed his eyes and leapt back down like someone suddenly awakening from a dream – and he saw that 'beyond the body there is a body', like a little child grown large. Yet not able to roam far, he speedily re-entered his mortal body; he re-entered and did not shed his form, matching his years with those of Heaven and earth. If he had 'shed his husk' and not re-entered in, he would have dwelt apart from this mortal world.

Mr Lu's method of shedding the Seven-Storied Jewelled Pagoda or Three-Stepped Red Building was much like that of Mr Zhong Li's.

But at his 'inner gazing', as the Imperial Chain-and-Bucket Water Pump scooped up his spirit to enter into the Heavenly Palace, he lingered, hankering after the clustered beauty of the scene – and thus unwittingly was transformed and shed out.

He raised a true fire and from within the smoke and flame transformed himself into a single Fire Dragon. Then he leapt out and away from the Dark Thoroughfare of this mortal life and achieved thus the extreme mystery of 'shedding his husk'.

Again our common ancestor and Zen Teacher (the Zen monk Master Mazu), although he made no use of the alchemical timing of the firing, was none the less able to scatter any Yin Magic; and with reference to 'inner gazing' and 'entering into settledness' he used the idea of a 'single spiritual chime' and departed. As he heard the sound of a stone hitting a tile, he at once transcended.[1] But he was only able to 'shed the husk' – he did not reveal the method of entering into the state of a Divine Immortal.

And also the Dharma's Sixth Patriarch and Zen Teacher, although he made Yin Magic, he 'shed his husk'. He first made the body like dried timber, and his heart like dead ashes. Then once he had assembled together the collected powers of his mind, with one intent, his understanding and thought inwardly protected, he stepped up from the heart region, clambering, step by step, to directly cross over the thirty-three heavens, and joyfully transform at the Heavenly Palace – just like the Daoists going to rest at the Upper Palace.

And then, bowing down at the point of approach, he took the Central Gate of the Three and 'shed his husk'. This was being able to 'shed' – but not being able to walk the Path.

In such a manner the Ancient Sages of the Western Mountain, once their task was complete and their life's work fulfilled, they shed their mortal husks. Even though they did not depart from 'inner

---

1   A famous Zen (Chan) tale.

gazing', they raised a fire, singing and playing, entering on in and passing on out through the gate.

To 'raise a fire' means to 'pole up the spirit to enter the crown', whilst to 'pass through the gate' is 'to refine and harmonise the spirit' and 'shed the husk'.

NOW WITH REFERENCE TO WHAT HAPPENS AFTER THE moment of 'inner gazing' and 'raising a fire', when thoughts arise like 'bustling flowers heavily laden', just think on a solitary village, and on a hut containing two or three rooms. Then you exit out but, 'hardly, hardly departed', you return to cast your eyes upon the 'Old Orchard', trusting in it being deserted and vacant…and on the point of your departure, not being able quite to achieve it, you return to look back and thus create the possibility of telling others about the Path. So then, without missing a step, the knowledge may be transmitted from sage to sage, and you are all able to 'shed the husk' without it creating any difficulty.

The famous poem goes:

> The work complete you hesitate
> At the Capital Gate where you shed the spirit,
> Clustered flowers
> Untangle in your body.
> And you return to cast your eyes
> Upon the Old Orchard,
> On the scene you love so well, until
> Amongst the clustering blooms, heavily laden,
> You find a solitary village-home!

NOTE: The rural idyll of the Chinese.

But alas indeed! Lesser scholars do not know of these ways. Unable to enter into 'settledness' and dealing in Yin Magic, they cannot shed the spirit. One day they miss their chance to enter through the Gate to the Sky and neither can they return back to their original bodies.

Now they are named 'corpses loosened into the world' and lead people, who want to learn, astray. They are deeply immersed in their ignorance. At them we may silently smile!

On the Refined Path, You May Walk in the Divine

They are few indeed who can abandon all thought of
their own lives and retain a purity of heart and mind!

THE PEOPLE OF THIS WORLD DO NOT AWAKEN TO THE
Grand Principle, and it is all because they take the spark from the stone
and the glare of the lightning in the sky as evidence of understanding
in this dusty world – and seek nourishment from them alone – which
means that, for a moment, from these outer sights, they find a crumb
of comfort. This is stated in *The Annals Recorded on the Vault of the Sky*.

They enslave the thread of their thoughts, winding it around and
around without ceasing, until one day their breath is weakened, and
they sicken and fall ill. Then their life-breath is cut off and they die,
caught in the transmigration of body and soul, without awakening.
And so the stream of the self re-assumes another form – they pass
on magically to another husk, and in the end are not free from the
succession of lives and deaths.

The real task is to rebuild and sustain the True Breath; once this
reality is rebuilt, then to forge and smelt out the Yang Spirit – and
then once the Yang Spirit has 'shed its husk', you may leave this

dusty world, and thenceforth dwell on the Three Isles of the Blest Immortals.

NOTE: This is the Daoist's ultimate goal.

The task complete, the spirit approaches the point of 'shedding its husk' – so now you must turn back to transmit your experience to the people of this world. Once this activity is complete and the whole task finished, you will receive a Royal Beckoning from the Celestial Lists, thenceforth to dwell unhindered in the Vault of the Sky.

Once you have found the Path, it is not possible to refuse to teach it. This is reported in *The Record on the Trickling Stream Finding a Path*. But teach it to the wrong person and misfortune will follow you down seven generations! And if you find the right person but avoid the teaching, then disaster will also befall your body.

The Sage of the Red Pines cautioned the Yellow Emperor, saying: 'The Way cannot be selfishly sought...'

It is necessary, in such a fashion, that people and creatures so progress. The principles of the Way demand a belief in the permanence of the Gold, the immutable spirit of humankind and a revelation of its unchanging aspect.

THE *WESTERN MOUNTAIN RECORDS* STATE THAT THE one who is granted this truth will manifest as one with a determined heart and mind: one who has been received on to the Path. The very greatest gifts are then bestowed upon their person and body, middling gifts upon their children and descendants, and the very least upon their neighbourhood and fields.

The very highest gifts that are bestowed include a Path for the people; the middling gifts include various methods for the people; the very least provide some minor tricks for the people to follow.

The True Sage 'Sprout' warns us that to pass on a knowledge of the Path to others, you must yearn to accompany the former Sages in their established destiny.

NOTE: The text draws to its conclusion
now with a strict admonishment.

Meeting with fellows of a determined heart and mind does not mean meeting with those who do not believe in the Gold or do not pass on its knowledge to others, and meeting with fellows of a determined mind does not mean meeting with those who believe in the Gold but do not vigorously promote it – for, if you do not make a special effort, it depletes the teaching and Path, and this is of benefit to no one.

The True Fellow 'Jade' questioned the True Master 'Silent Virtue' saying: The best of those amongst the Immortals entered into the Southern Isles, but yet passed on to us the destiny of the Path. I want to make a sworn covenant to follow them, so how do I do it?

Then the True Master replied, saying: Now the men of the Southern Isles were dripping in blessings and happiness! If you do not believe in the Workings of Heaven, but take your life lightly and concentrate on mere possessions, truly you will become a low-down ghost or devil. If you do not establish a belief in the Eternal Gold, others will twist about your thinking. If you do not make a sworn covenant with the Ancient Sages, others will decry you and your powers slip away.

Therefore acquire knowledge through pondering the Eternal Gold – and through finding a way to display its unchanging aspect.

Oh, alas indeed! The people of this world throng about us. But not one of them has an aspiring heart, silent and clear; and amongst ten thousand, silent and clear, there is not one with a determined heart and mind; and amongst ten thousand with a determined heart and mind there is not one bright enough and perceptive enough to penetrate the Workings of Heaven and think little of wealth and possessions.

Those who can abandon all thought of their own lives and retain a purity of heart and mind are few!

In general people assume the Path whilst seeking for gain and possessions; through lying and deceit they may become scholars of a determined mind, but they catch sight of the Noble Path and then abandon it. Consequently when they employ students, they bind their hands and gag their mouths. In the end they all confront death together, and cannot be aided!

If you are a scholar who promotes this Path, who can understand others and tell the stupid from the wise, who has received instruction in the methods – and knows the correct way to set about them – then after a long period of time and practice you will acquire some skill and get results.

This will produce a 'glorious florescence' that is the mark of the Gold – and this Gold has a worth beyond anything you could ever repay to your former friends and teachers. Just be thankful.

> *NOTE: Herein is displayed the true aspect of our internal nature, the revelation of the permanence and glory of our Golden Selves, as true as any imperishable treasure. We need to teach others how we may all be alive and akin to the True Breath of Heaven and earth.*

GLOSSARY

Individuals

TEACHER LU, DUKE LU, MR LU Lü Tung-Pin; born 796, Shi Jianwu's spiritual teacher.

OUR GENTLEMAN IMMORTAL, LORD GE IMMORTAL A title for Ge Hong (283–343 CE) literary scholar, philosopher and alchemist from the Western Jin. Tradition states he 'shed his husk' and attained immortality.

HUA TUO Eastern Han physician, died 208 CE.

ZHEN YI Possibly the Zhen Yi mentioned in the *Zhuangzi*, fourth century BCE ('Kings who Resign' chapter).

MASTER GUANG ZHENG, OLD MASTER ZHENG Legendary teacher of the Yellow Emperor.

YELLOW EMPEROR Legendary founder of traditional Chinese medicine.

LAO ZI Earliest Daoist philosopher (sixth century BCE?), legendary author of *Tao-te Ching*.

BODHIDHARMA Fifth-century Buddhist monk, legendary transmitter of Zen (Chan) Buddhism to China.

BIAN QUE One of the most famous ancient Chinese physicians, died 310 BCE, said to have authored or commentated on the *Lingshu* medical classic.

LIUDONG Unknown, may be a contemporary figure.

MASTER FROM THE RED PINES, SAGE OF THE RED PINES Legendary figure from the Qin and Han dynasties.

TRUE MASTER 'PROPER UNITY' Possibly Zhang Ling, a nebulous Daoist from the Han dynasty.

TRUE LORD YIN Lived during the Han dynasty, mentioned by Ge Hong.

'FREELY WANDERING' MASTER Not clear who this is; the term 'freely wandering' first occurs in the *Zhuangzi*.

FANG-TAN Unidentified.

QIAN-SAN Unidentified.

'WATERY TOAD', MASTER 'SEA TOAD' A renowned and contemporary patriarch of internal alchemy, much revered during later centuries.

MR WANG Unknown.

KING LIU Also known as Liu Anwang, King of Huainan, who, very early on, used boiled-up and distilled urine to create the first steroid hormonal pill. This is described in the *Huainan Zi* (second century BCE).

TRUE MAN LIU GANG Eastern Han official, part-time Daoist and pursuer of immortality.

TRUE FELLOW 'SUPREME PURITY', 'GREAT WHITE' OR 'GREAT PURITY', LI BAI Famous Tang dynasty poet (701–762), also known as Li Bo.

BREAKING BRIGHT DAWN An elderly adept, probably a contemporary figure.

MR ZHONG LI One of 'eight Daoist Immortals'.

MASTER MAZU Influential eighth-century Zen monk, known for his forthright manner.

DHARMA'S SIXTH PATRIARCH Huineng (638–713), Sixth Patriarch of Zen (Chan) Buddhism in China.

Terms

FIVE CONSTANTS, FIVE VAPOURS, FIVE CYCLES OF FORM Water, fire, wood, earth and metal/gold, the so-called Five Elements.

TRUE BREATH Real, self-sustaining, donated to us by Heaven and earth; not the coarse 'worldly' breath.

TWO BREATHS Yin and Yang.

THREE POWERS Heaven, Man and Earth.

DAOYIN A physical method of conducting *qi*-energy, stretching exercises.

THREE FLOWERS The fluid-essences, breath and spirit (*jing, qi* and *shen*).

TRUE LEAD AND TRUE MERCURY The True Yin and True Yang.

TRUE LEAD Resilient and unchanging. Zhang Boduan (Song dynasty alchemist and poet, founder of the Southern School) says, 'silver moonlight… shining at the end of the day on Western River', that is, light hidden within water. Again, see the great poet Su Dongpo…'the river streams past, but is never gone, the moon waxes and wanes but remains' from his 'Red Cliff Ode'.

YELLOW SPROUT The birth of the Yang spirit.

PROPER YANG In this text, most often the vapour of the Proper Yang, the Yang Dragon.

LI-FIRE, QIAN-HEAVEN, KAN-WATER, GEN-MOUNTAIN, SUN-WIND, KUN-EARTH, ZHEN-THUNDER, DUI-MARSH The eight trigrams of the *Yijing*.

DANTIAN 'Cinnabar Field', 'elixial field', also named 'lower field', close to acupoint Ren.6.

JIA-YI, GENG-XIN Pairs of 'Heavenly Stems', relate to rising and falling, dawn and dusk, opening and close.

HUN-SOUL, PO-SOUL Reside in the liver and lungs, respectively.

SILENT SOURCE My translation of *yuan* 元 ('originating, primary, life affirming').

HEXAGRAM, TRIGRAM A six-line or three-line figure from the *Yijing*.

TRUE MEDICINE The true Yin and Yang born in the body, true in two senses: *ideal*, but also *real*, the natural goodness in each man and woman, our 'higher nature', self-affirming, a link to Heaven and earth. Thus 'without the body there is another body, whereby we may transcend earthly matters to walk in the divine'.

Book titles (selective)

The Secret Book of Our Father Probably Lao Zi's *Tao-te Ching*.

Tao-te Ching The Book of the Way and its Power, first classic of Daoism, attributed to Lao Zi (literally, the 'old boy').

Lingshu The Spiritual Pivot, the first book on acupuncture; it has been attributed to Bian Que.

The Book of the Matching Shadow Possibly eighth-century Daoist scripture, enormously influential.

Yijing One of the oldest books in the world, and classic of Chinese literature – written to give explicit knowledge of how to conform with 'human nature and life's innermost pattern' (*xing ming*). It uses *gua* symbolism (hexagrams and trigrams) to explain both the physical and spiritual aspects of nature. For instance, Kan may stand for water, kidneys, heaviness, winter, cooling, etc. whilst Li represents fire, the heart, lightness, heating, the summer, etc.